Acquired Cystic Disease of the Kidney and Renal Cell Carcinoma
Complications of Long-Term Dialysis

Isao Ishikawa

Acquired Cystic Disease of the Kidney and Renal Cell Carcinoma

Complications of Long-Term Dialysis

With 144 Figures, Including 122 in Color

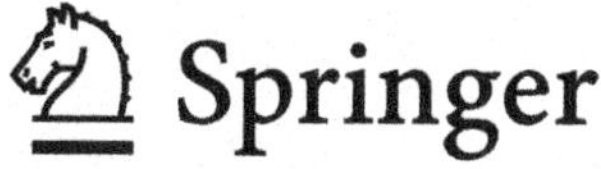 Springer

Isao Ishikawa, M.D.
Emeritus Professor, Kanazawa Medical University
1-35 Kohyo-Dai, Uchinada, Kahoku, Ishikawa 920-0272, Japan;
Division of Nephrology, Asanogawa General Hospital
83 Kosaka-Naka, Kanazawa, Ishikawa 920-8621, Japan

ISBN 978-4-431-56319-8 Springer Tokyo Berlin Heidelberg New York
DOI 10.1007/978-4-431-69481-6

Springer is a part of Springer Science+Business Media
springer.com
© Springer 2007
Softcover re-print of the Hardcover 1st edition 2007

Typesetting: SNP Best-set Typesetter Ltd., Hong Kong
Printing and binding: Shinano, Inc., Japan

Preface

I have been involved in the treatment of chronic renal insufficiency for 40 years, beginning with peritoneal dialysis immediately after graduation from medical school in 1965, then with hemodialysis in 1967 after I first experienced it in Kanazawa, and with renal transplantation since 1972, when I was studying in the United States. During this period, the number of dialysis patients has continued to increase rapidly to the present figure of 257 765 (at the end of 2005), and with surprising increases in the survival rate. However, new and unexpected pathological conditions have also appeared as complications of long-term dialysis. One of these involves polycystic changes and their malignant transformation in diseased kidneys. Since I have studied these polycystic changes and their malignant transformation for many years, I decided to compile the results of my work in a book. Such conditions of diseased kidneys pose serious problems, particularly in Japan, where renal transplantation is performed very infrequently compared with other countries, and a large number of patients are managed by dialysis over a long period.

Contents

Summary of Acquired Cystic Disease of the Kidney and Renal Cell Carcinoma

1. Diseased kidneys shrink for 3 years after the initiation of dialysis, but enlarge thereafter due to the development of acquired renal cysts with an associated increase in the risk of renal cell carcinoma (see front cover). However, successful renal transplantation results in a gradual regression of cysts, a shrinking of diseased kidneys, and a decrease in the risk of renal cell carcinoma. Unfortunately, this effect may be somewhat attenuated by immunosuppressants and further evaluation is necessary (Fig. 1).

2. The incidence of renal cell carcinoma is higher in dialysis patients than in the general population. Among dialysis patients, the risk of renal cell carcinoma is higher in males, in those with a longer history of dialysis, and in those with more severe cystic changes. In addition, as renal cell carcinomas are related to cysts, there is often a papillary renal tumor, with a possible multistep progress from cysts to adenoma and then to renal cell carcinoma. A renal cell carcinoma surrounded by cysts is difficult to diagnose. Although the prognosis is generally good, caution is necessary

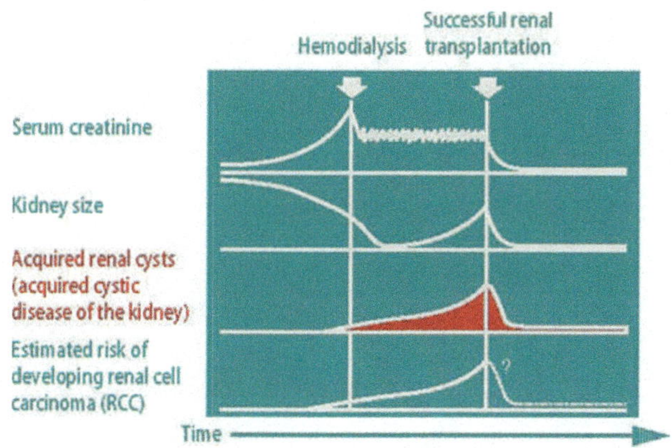

FIG. 1. Relationship between the condition of chronic renal failure (serum creatinine), kidney size, number of acquired cysts, and the estimated risk of renal cell carcinoma (Reproduced from [14], with permission from Elsevier Inc.)

because of metastasis and rapid tumor growth in some patients. Double cancers are also frequently observed.

3. Renal cell carcinoma is an important complication of long-term dialysis, but screening is necessary for diagnosis because it occurs frequently and is asymptomatic. However, screening all dialysis patients is not reasonable from a cost-effect viewpoint. Whether or not a patient should be screened must be evaluated on an individual basis. Screening is necessary in high-risk patients and before all renal transplantations.

4. Since very few renal transplantations are performed in Japan, a very large number of patients are receiving long-term dialysis. Patients with a high risk of developing renal cell carcinoma must be screened periodically, except for those who would not tolerate surgery.

Chapter 1
Beginning the Research

In 1978, a 24-year-old man who had been managed by hemodialysis for 7 years was referred to our department for emergency nephrectomy as his "autosomal dominant polycystic kidney disease" was infected, and the condition had become uncontrollable (Fig. 2). A large hematoma was present in the resected lower pole of the right kidney, and multiple small cysts were observed in both kidneys. The pathology department reported autosomal dominant polycystic kidney disease (ADPKD) complicated by hematoma (Fig. 3). However, careful inquiry into the patient's history revealed that he had undergone renal biopsy 7 months before the initiation of dialysis, and had been diagnosed as having rapidly progressive glomerulonephritis (Figs. 4 and 5). This reminded me of something I had learned in 1972 while I was studying in the United States: "Cysts eventually develop in all end-stage kidneys." Reviewing the literature from that time, I came across an autopsy report by Dunnill et al. [1] (Fig. 6) published in 1977. This described cysts complicated by renal cell carcinoma (RCC). I therefore speculated that our patient had initially had rapidly progressive glomerulonephritis and thereafter had developed acquired renal cysts, which were then complicated by renal cell carcinoma, and that the hematoma was due to bleeding of the renal cell carcinoma. I requested that the pathology department reevaluate the case. The reevaluation disclosed a papillary renal cell carcinoma consisting of a clear cell carcinoma and a granular cell carcinoma on the hematoma wall (Fig. 7). This was my first clinical case of acquired cystic disease of the kidney and renal cell carcinoma, and also the first case in the world. This patient had developed bladder cancer 6 years earlier, had been treated, and as of September 2006, he is still in good health.

My research started with this clinical case in December 1978, when there were only 27 048 dialysis patients in Japan. Fortunately, this discovery coincided with the introduction of a computed tomography (CT) scanner to a hospital affiliated to our department in 1978–1979. We performed a CT scan on 96 patients at the affiliated hospital in order to examine their kidney size and discover whether they had any cysts or tumors. These patients (mean age 40 years) had all received replacement therapy for chronic glomerulonephritis, for a mean period of 3 years and 4 months. This study showed that diseased kidneys shrink for 3 years after the initiation of dialysis, but some of them begin to enlarge thereafter due to multiple cyst formation. Thus, the conventional idea that diseased kidneys remain atrophic even after the initiation

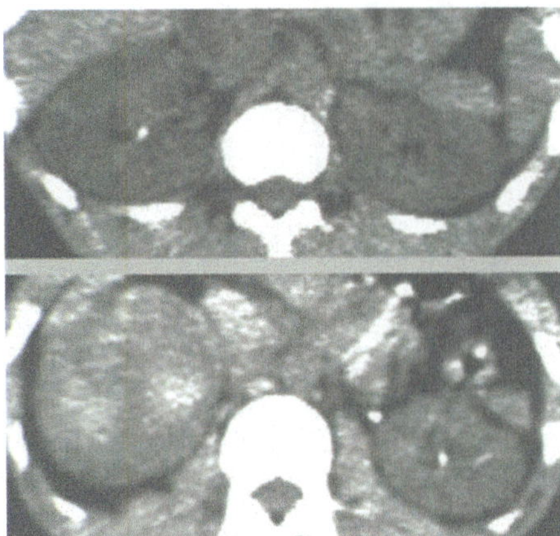

Fig. 2. Computed tomography (CT) images of the world's first clinical case. A large number of small cysts can be seen. *Above.* Acquired cystic disease of the kidney. *Below.* A mass and a hematoma are suspected in the right kidney

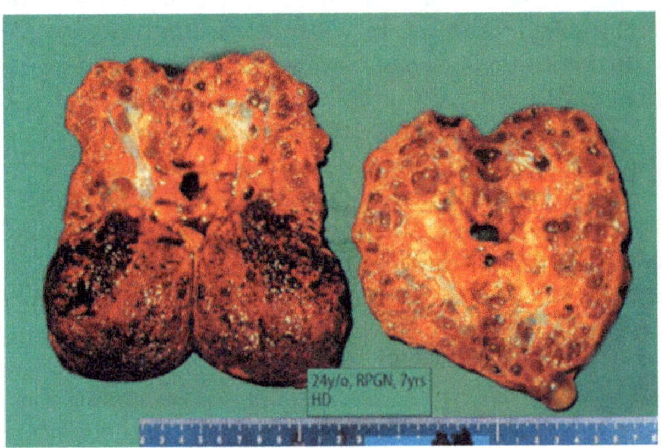

Fig. 3. Resected kidney. The world's first clinical case of acquired cystic disease of the kidney complicated by renal cell carcinoma

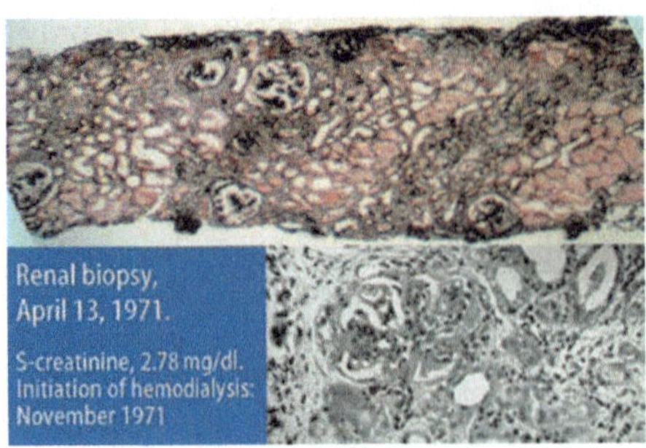

Fig. 4. Renal biopsy findings before the initiation of dialysis. *Above.* No cyst suggestive of autosomal dominant polycystic kidney disease was noted. *Below.* The findings indicated rapidly progressive glomerulonephritis

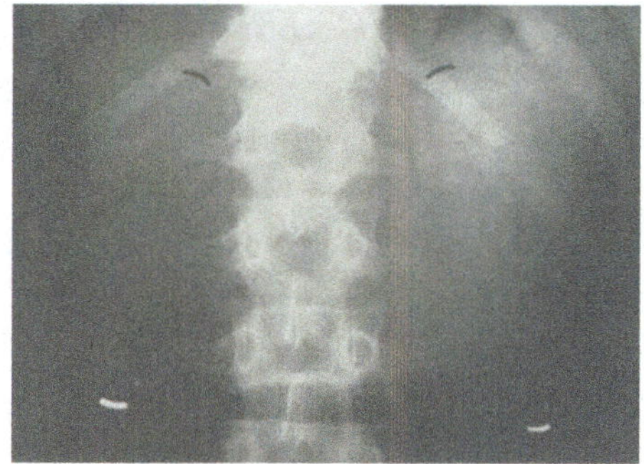

FIG. 5. Intravenous pyelogram (IVP) just before renal biopsy. The kidney size was normal or slightly large. The findings were not consistent with those of autosomal dominant polycystic kidney disease

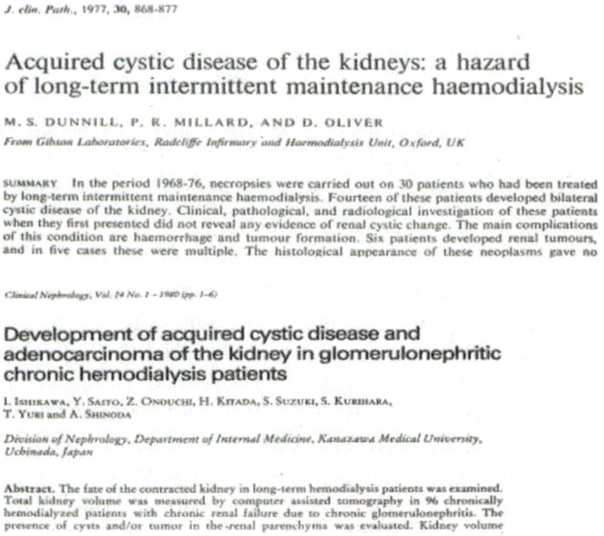

J. clin. Path., 1977, **30**, 868-877

Acquired cystic disease of the kidneys: a hazard of long-term intermittent maintenance haemodialysis

M. S. DUNNILL, P. R. MILLARD, AND D. OLIVER

From Gibson Laboratories, Radcliffe Infirmary and Haemodialysis Unit, Oxford, UK

SUMMARY In the period 1968-76, necropsies were carried out on 30 patients who had been treated by long-term intermittent maintenance haemodialysis. Fourteen of these patients developed bilateral cystic disease of the kidney. Clinical, pathological, and radiological investigation of these patients when they first presented did not reveal any evidence of renal cystic change. The main complications of this condition are haemorrhage and tumour formation. Six patients developed renal tumours, and in five cases these were multiple. The histological appearance of these neoplasms gave no

Clinical Nephrology, Vol. 14 No. 1 – 1980 (pp. 1–6)

Development of acquired cystic disease and adenocarcinoma of the kidney in glomerulonephritic chronic hemodialysis patients

I. Ishikawa, Y. Saito, Z. Onouchi, H. Kitada, S. Suzuki, S. Kurihara, T. Yuri and A. Shinoda

Division of Nephrology, Department of Internal Medicine, Kanazawa Medical University, Uchinada, Japan

Abstract. The fate of the contracted kidney in long-term hemodialysis patients was examined. Total kidney volume was measured by computer assisted tomography in 96 chronically hemodialyzed patients with chronic renal failure due to chronic glomerulonephritis. The presence of cysts and/or tumor in the renal parenchyma was evaluated. Kidney volume

FIG. 6. Titles of papers by Dunnill et al. and Ishikawa et al.

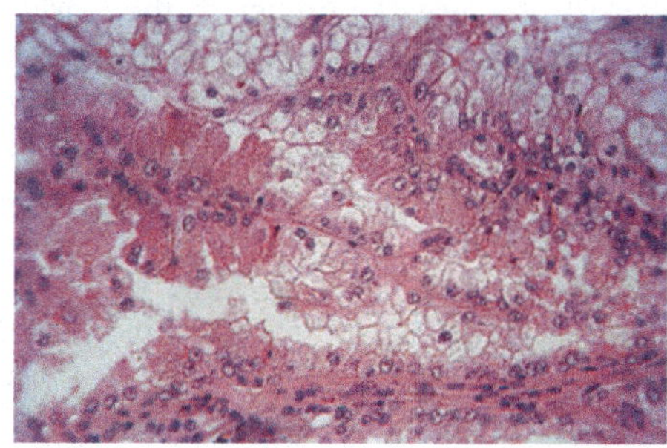

FIG. 7. Renal pathology. Papillary renal cell carcinoma in the hematoma wall consisting of clear and granular cells

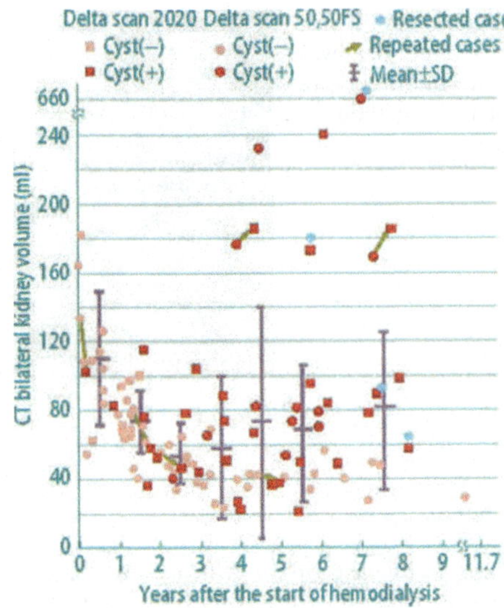

FIG. 8. Relationship of the duration of dialysis with the kidney volume and the presence or absence of cysts in 96 patients receiving dialysis for end-stage renal failure due to chronic glomerulonephritis (Reproduced from [2], with permission from Dustri-Verlag Dr. Karl Feistle)

of dialysis was found to be incorrect (Fig. 8). Furthermore, this screening disclosed the presence of renal cell carcinomas in two patients and adenoma in a patient (Fig. 8). An article describing these results was submitted to *Clinical Nephrology* in 1979, and was published in 1980 (Fig. 6) [2].

This finding that the diseased kidneys of dialysis patients develop acquired polycystic disease, and occasionally even renal cell carcinoma, was recognized as being very interesting in that it indicated a close relationship between renal cysts and renal cell carcinoma. In addition, since cell proliferation is indispensable for cyst development in autosomal dominant polycystic kidney disease, and since cysts are fluid-secreting neoplasms [3], the finding attracted the attention of cancer researchers as a human model of the multistep development of renal cell carcinoma, i.e., cysts→ adenoma→cancer.

In Japan, 96.3% of patients with end-stage renal disease are treated by hemodialysis, with the largest number in the world of relatively young patients undergoing long-term dialysis. Therefore, research in Japan into this complication of long-term dialysis has gained global recognition [4–8].

Chapter 2
Acquired Cystic Disease of the Kidney

The designation of "acquired cystic disease of the kidney": This disease is called "acquired cystic disease of the kidney," "acquired renal cystic disease," or "acquired cystic kidney disease" in the English-language literature. However, I considered that these terms did not truly represent the characteristics of the disease and named it *ta-nouhouka-isyukujin* in Japanese, thus implying that atrophic kidneys later develop multiple renal cysts [9]. At present, the terms *ta-nouhouka-isyukujin* in Japanese, ACDK, and "acquired cystic disease of the kidney" are used in Japan, of which the first two are predominant.

1 Definition of Acquired Cystic Disease of the Kidney

The term "acquired cystic disease of the kidney" means a condition in which acquired multiple cysts develop in the atrophied bilateral kidneys regardless of the primary disease [10,11]. While the incidence of the disease is not related to age [12], cystic changes tend to be more severe in younger patients [13]. In relation to specific diagnostic criteria, a condition in which 3–5 cysts are found in one kidney by imaging studies is clinically diagnosed as acquired cystic disease of the kidney (ACDK) [2,14–18]. However, there have been reports that about 20 cysts were found in a pathological examination when only 1 cyst had been found by imaging studies [2,19], and therefore a condition in which one cyst or more is observed in the bilateral kidneys may be defined as ACDK [2]. The diagnostic criteria can vary according to the subjects and the purpose of the research, but a pathological diagnosis is made when between 25% [20] and 40% [21] or more of a renal cross section is occupied by cysts.

2 Prevalence

Concerning the relationship between the duration of dialysis therapy and the prevalence of cystic changes, cysts have been observed in 12% of patients before the initiation of dialysis. Their prevalence increases progressively with the duration of dialysis: 44% after less than 3 years, 79% after 3 years or longer, 90% after 10 years or longer, and 93% after 20 years or longer [11] (Fig. 9).

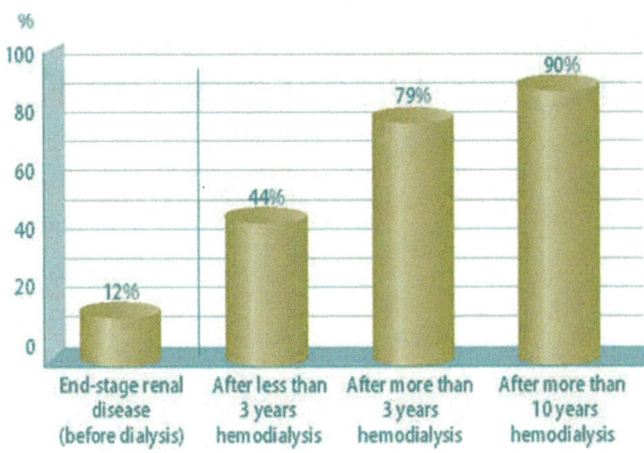

FIG. 9. Duration of dialysis and the prevalence of acquired cystic disease of the kidney

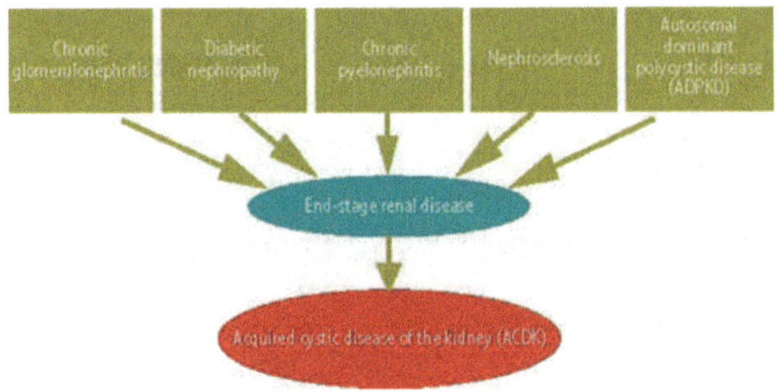

FIG. 10. Relationship between autosomal dominant polycystic kidney disease (ADPKD) and acquired cystic disease of the kidney (ACDK)

3 Primary Disease

I consider that ACDK occurs regardless of the primary disease, and that it may also occur in autosomal dominant polycystic kidney disease (ADPKD). However, I have the impression that the development of cysts is delayed in diabetic nephropathy [22], and that there are fewer cysts in hypoplastic kidneys. Figure 10 shows the relationships between primary diseases and ACDK.

4 Histology of Acquired Cystic Disease of the Kidney

With ACDK, the weight of the bilateral kidneys combined is often 20–300 g, but one kidney may weigh as much as 1250 g [20] and attain a size which is indistinguishable from those found in ADPKD [23].

FIG. 11. A macroscopic cross section of a kidney with acquired cystic disease of the kidney (transverse section, CT cut). Although small cysts were observed in large numbers, only one cyst in the upper middle area could be diagnosed by imaging techniques. The other cysts were difficult to delineate (Reproduced from [11], with permission from S. Karger AG)

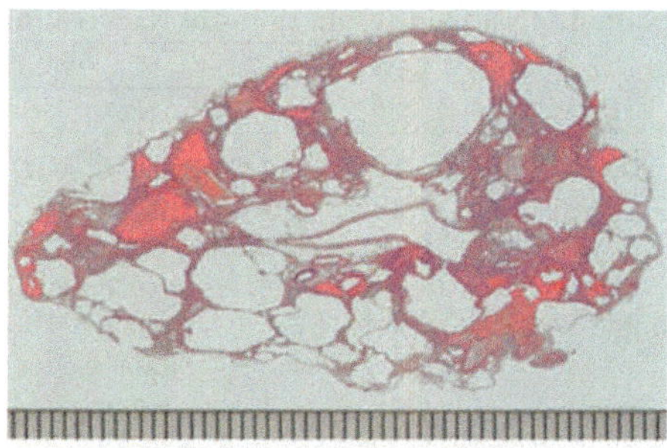

FIG. 12. Scanning electron microscopy of the cyst wall. The cyst epithelium has a brush border and shows the characteristics of the proximal tubules

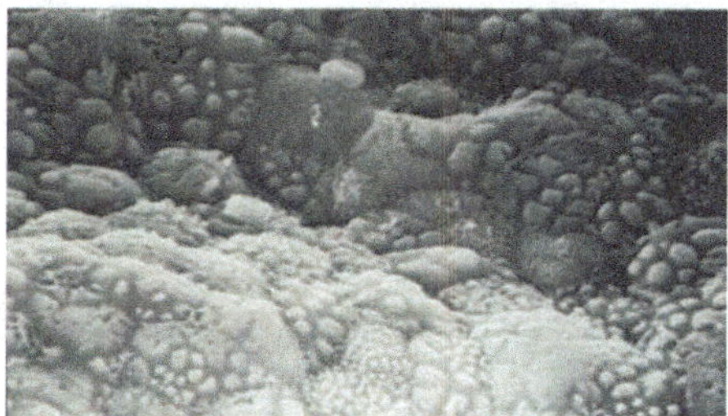

Figure 11 shows a cross section of a kidney with ACDK. Most of the renal parenchyma has been replaced by cysts. Many of the cysts are small, with a diameter of 0.02–2 cm, and 94% of them are 0.6 cm or less in diameter [19,24]. The pathological features indicating the sequence cysts→adenoma→renal cell carcinoma, as reported by Dunnill et al. [1], are also often noted. Renal cell carcinoma is often observed in dialysis patients because it frequently occurs with ACDK due to its relationship with cysts, and dialysis patients often have ACDK. In other words, a histological characteristic of ACDK is epithelial hyperplasia (a high proliferation ability of cyst epithelium), which suggests a precancerous condition. In addition, the kidney becomes larger as there are more renal cysts with high proliferation ability, and the risk of renal cell carcinoma is higher as the kidney becomes larger due to cysts.

A study of the course of the development of cysts in early lesions showed that acquired renal cysts begin to develop in young patients aged less than 50 years while the glomerular filtration rate (GFR) remains between 52 and 71 ml/min [25].

5 Origin of Cysts

On scanning electron microscopy, the brush border can be observed on the cyst epithelium (Fig. 12). In ACDK, the cyst fluid/serum ratio is 1.0 for Na, high at 5–7 for creatinine, but abnormally low at 0.06 for β_2-microglobulin, and the concentrations of these factors are in agreement with those in tubular fluid in the distal part of the proximal tubules [26,27] (Table 1). Therefore, cysts of ACDK are considered to originate from proximal tubules. Moreover, the following findings also suggest that the proximal tubules are the origins of cysts. On immunological staining using lectin,

TABLE 1. Cyst fluid/serum ratios of Na, creatinine, and β_2-microglobulin

	Case	Cyst fluid/serum ratio		
		Na	Creatinine	β_2 microglobulin
ACDK	1	1.096 ± 0.036* (7)**	7.058 ± 1.311 (7)	0.053 ± 0.057 (7)
	2	1.087 ± 0.027 (10)	5.363 ± 1.369 (10)	0.060 ± 0.022 (8)
	3	1.038 ± 0.012 (9)	6.855 ± 1.465 (9)	0.004 ± 0.008 (7)
	mean	1.07 ± 0.036 (26)	6.332 ± 1.581 (26)	0.040 ± 0.008 (22)
Simple cysts	4	1.075	0.867	1.864
	5	1.077	1.000	0.846
	6	1.109	1.375	
	mean	1.087 ± 0.019 (3)	1.081 ± 0.263 (3)	1.355 (2)
ADPKD	7	1.007	0.843	—

*, Mean ± SD; **, Number of cysts; ACDK, acquired cystic disease of the kidney; ADPKD, autosomal dominant polycystic kidney disease

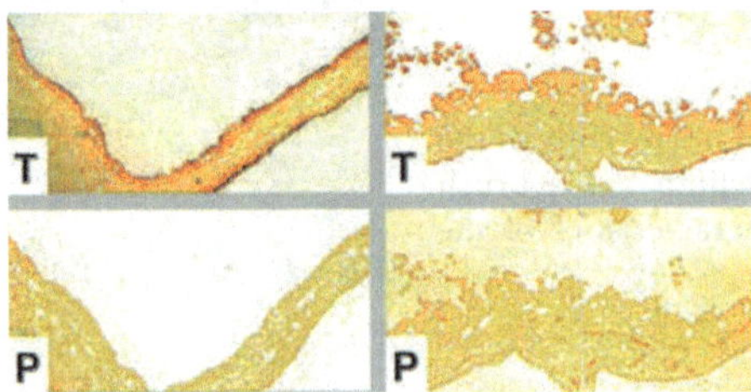

FIG. 13. Lectin immunological staining. On lectin staining of the monolayer epithelium (*left*) and the multilayer cyst epithelium (atypical cyst) (*right*), tetragonolobus (*T*) was positive (+), and peanut lectin (*P*) was negative (–), indicating the proximal tubular origin of the tumor (Reproduced from [28], with permission from S. Karger AG)

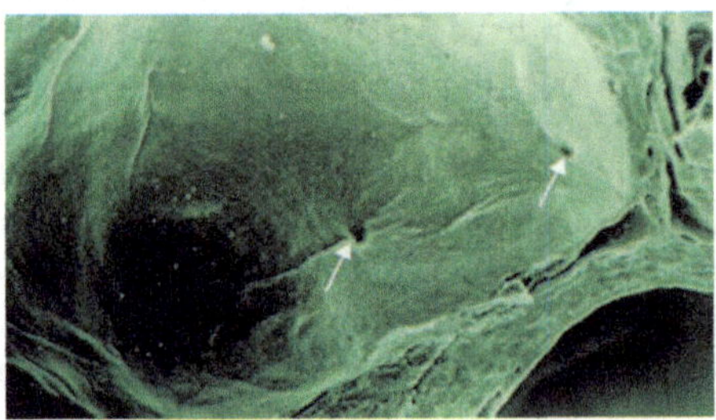

FIG. 14. Scanning electron microscopy. Holes (*arrows*) suggestive of communication with renal tubules can be seen on the wall surface of acquired renal cysts

tetragonolobus lectin, indicating the proximal tubules, is positive, but peanut lectin, indicating the distal tubules, is negative [28] (Fig. 13), paraaminohippuric acid is excreted into the cyst fluid [29], and intramuscularly administered gentamicin is recovered from the cyst fluid [29]. In addition, cysts communicating with renal tubules are observed more frequently in ACDK than in simple renal cysts or in ADPKD [30] (Fig. 14).

6 Complications of Acquired Cystic Disease of the Kidney

While the incidence of ACDK is high, there is no clinical problem unless there are any of the first four of the following five complications: (1) renal cell carcinoma; (2) retroperitoneal bleeding; (3) renal abscess; (4) protein stones [17]; (5) a high hematocrit. Among these complications, renal cell carcinoma and retroperitoneal bleeding due to cyst rupture are particularly serious. Figure 15 shows computed tomography (CT) scans of a massive hemorrhage caused by a ruptured cyst.

6.1 Renal Cell Carcinoma

Renal cell carcinoma is discussed in Chapter 3.

6.2 Retroperitoneal Bleeding

Prevalence. The cases of retroperitoneal bleeding were reported by Tuttle et al. and others [31–33]. From our experience, we consider that its prevalence is about 0.5%, or one-third of that of renal cell carcinoma. I have encountered 10 cases of this condition [10,34].

Risk. There are considered to be four main risk factors for retroperitoneal bleeding: (1) male sex; (2) enlargement of the kidney due to marked cystic changes with long-term dialysis therapy; (3) use of anticoagulants; (4) mechanical stress such as coughing.

Symptoms. Retroperitoneal bleeding must be considered first if a patient exhibits symptoms such as sudden shock, a decrease in blood pressure, loin pain, lateral

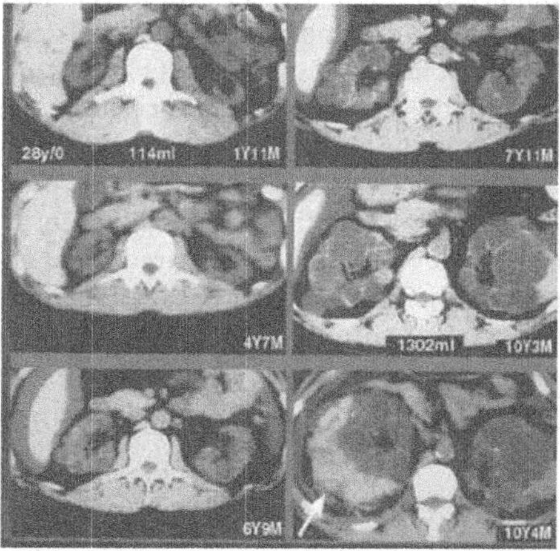

FIG. 15. Retroperitoneal bleeding due to rupture of an acquired renal cyst (*arrow*). Images of a continuous ambulatory peritoneal dialysis (CAPD) patient (Reproduced from [34], with permission from Elsevier Inc.)

abdominal pain, or nausea/vomiting after mechanical stress such as coughing while the patient is still under the influence of an anticoagulant after dialysis.

Diagnosis. A CT scan is the most reliable way to diagnose retroperitoneal bleeding. It should be performed first, because it allows an estimation of the volume of the hemorrhage as well as confirming the diagnosis of retroperitoneal bleeding.

Mechanism of bleeding. Bleeding appears to be caused by the rupture of an artery in the cyst wall [31]. Retroperitoneal bleeding includes bleeding from a renal cell carcinoma occurring in the cyst wall or developing as a mass.

Treatment. The patient should first be treated conservatively by a blood transfusion. If the blood pressure cannot be maintained even after the transfusion of 1000 ml blood, renal artery embolization or nephrectomy should be performed. However, even if conservative therapy has been successful, continued observation is important because about 30% of patients with retroperitoneal bleeding have renal cell carcinoma [20].

6.3 Renal Abscess

We reported the first case of renal abscess as a complication of ACDK in 1980 [35], but we have seen only a few cases since then, and few are reported in the literature; renal abscess is a rare complication of ACDK.

6.4 Protein Stones

Although Mickisch et al. [17] described protein stones as a complication of ACDK, it is presently considered to be unrelated to the complications or causes of ACDK.

6.5 Increase in Hematocrit

Because anemia is mild in autosomal dominant polycystic kidney disease (ADPKD), there is a very attractive hypothesis that the hematocrit increases as acquired renal cysts develop. I have doubts as to whether this hypothesis is valid, because anemia is reported to be alleviated with the development of acquired renal cysts in about half of the articles published, but not in the remaining half [14]. According to our research, no increases in serum erythropoietin concentration or hematocrit were observed with increases in cysts [36]. Moreover, the hematocrit increased while the kidneys remained small in some patients on long-term dialysis therapy, and some female patients did not develop cysts but showed an alleviation of anemia even on long-term dialysis. The relationship between the development of acquired renal cysts and an improvement in the hematocrit is now difficult to clarify because anemic patients are rare due to the use of erythropoietin (rHuEpo).

7 Characteristics of Acquired Cystic Disease of the Kidney

7.1 Prevalence Increases with Duration of Dialysis

The prevalence of ACDK is closely related to the duration of dialysis and, as mentioned above, is 44% when the duration of dialysis is less than 3 years, but reaches 79% when dialysis lasts for 3 years or longer [2].

7.2 Sex Differences

Cystic changes in the kidney occur more frequently and are more severe in males than in females [37] (Fig. 16). Figure 17 shows the CT scans of two patients, both of whom had a 14-year history of hemodialysis. While many cysts can be seen in the male patient, few can be seen in the female patient. We started a follow-up study of diseased kidneys in 96 dialysis patients in 1979. After 10 years, the mean kidney

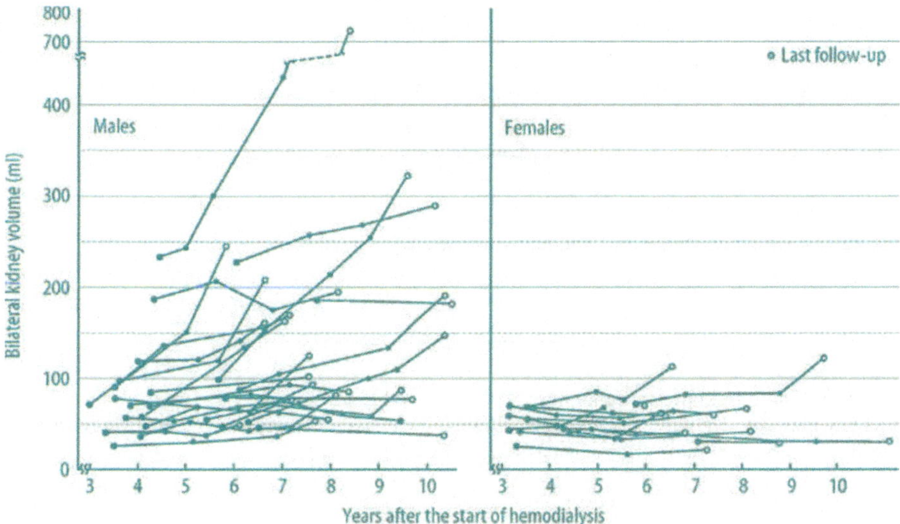

FIG. 16. Sex differences in the kidney volume in acquired cystic disease of the kidney. Cystic changes are more prevalent and more severe in males (Reproduced from [37], with permission from S. Karger AG)

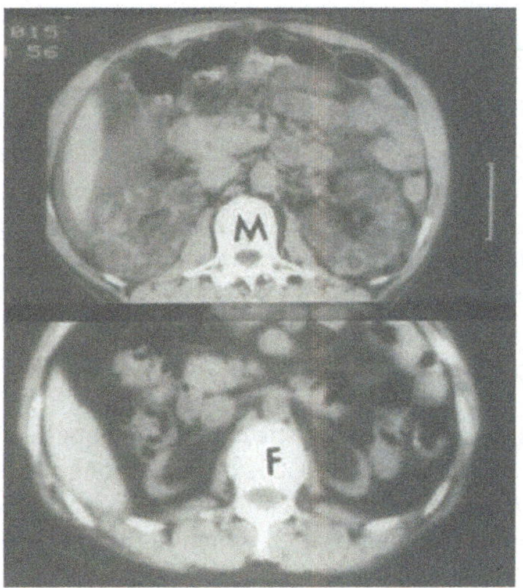

FIG. 17. Sex differences in acquired cystic disease of the kidney. Cystic changes were more severe in the male (*M*) than in the female (*F*), both of whom had a 14-year history of dialysis

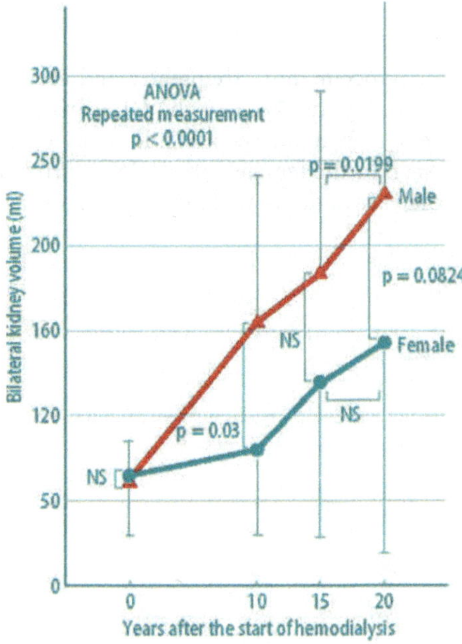

FIG. 18. Changes in kidney volume over 20 years. The kidney volume was larger in male than in female patients. An increase in kidney volume indicates the occurrence of cysts (Reproduced from [13], with permission from Dustri-Verlag Dr. Karl Feistle)

volume had increased 2.7 times from 81 ml to 207 ml in males, but had increased only 1.5 times from 66 ml to 86 ml in females [34,38,39]. Sex differences were also observed in my 20-year follow-up study, where the kidney volume differed between males and females after 15 years [40] and 20 years [13] (Fig. 18).

7.3 Dialysis Modality

The prevalence of cystic changes is not affected by the dialysis modality [38,39]. A comparison among dialysis modalities showed that the incidence of cystic changes was similar between continuous ambulatory peritoneal dialysis (CAPD) and hemo-dialysis [41] (Fig. 19). Figure 15 shows CT scans of a 28-year-old man treated by CAPD after having undergone hemodialysis for 5 years. Cystic changes are known to occur under management by CAPD as they do with hemodialysis.

7.4 Dialyzer Membrane

The incidence of cystic changes is not affected by the dialyzer. We examined whether the incidence of ACDK differs among types of dialyzer. No difference was observed between cellulose membranes, which are reported to markedly activate cytokines, and synthetic membranes, which do not [42] (Fig. 20).

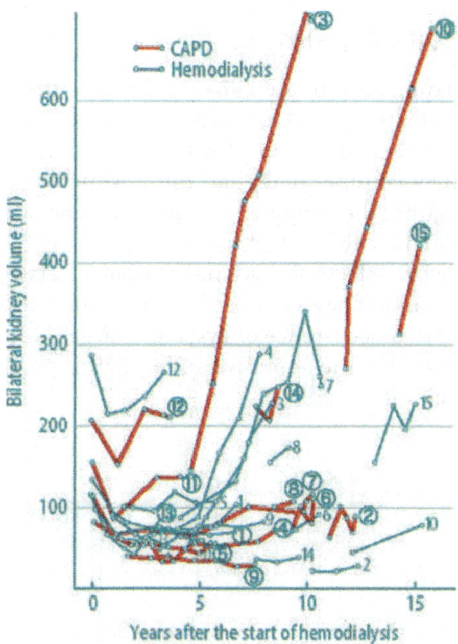

Fig. 19. Comparison of the occurrence of acquired renal cysts (acquired cystic disease of the kidney) in CAPD patients and hemodialysis patients. Paired cases are indicated by the same numbers (Reproduced from [41], with permission from Multimed Inc.)

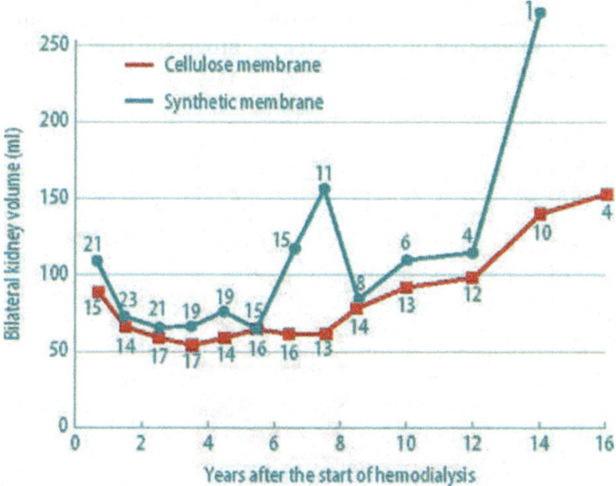

Fig. 20. Comparison of kidney volume between patients who received dialysis using a dialyzer with a cellulosic membrane and those who received dialysis using a dialyzer with a synthetic membrane. No differences in the kidney volume were observed. The numbers in the figure indicate the number of cases

7.5 Relationship with Erythropoietin

Figure 21 shows the relationships of the kidney volume to the serum erythropoietin concentration and the hematocrit. There was no difference in either the erythropoietin concentration or the hematocrit between the patients who showed a 2-fold or greater increase in kidney volume (blue) and those who showed a smaller increase (red) [36]. Therefore, neither the serum erythropoietin concentration nor the hematocrit was higher in patients with marked cystic changes.

Next, we examined what effects the administration of erythropoietin (rHuEpo) exerts on cystic changes or kidney volume. We found that this treatment was not associated with an increased occurrence of cysts or a larger kidney volume [43] (Fig. 22). Therefore, I speculate that the administration of rHuEpo does not promote the growth of renal cell carcinoma.

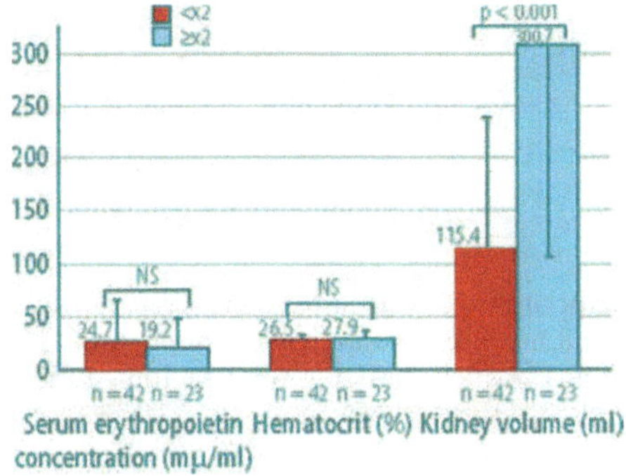

FIG. 21. Comparisons of changes in the serum erythropoietin concentration and hematocrit between a group with a 2-fold increase in kidney volume or more and a group with a less than 2-fold increase during a 10-year period. Neither the erythropoietin level nor the hematocrit was higher in the group that showed a marked increase in cysts

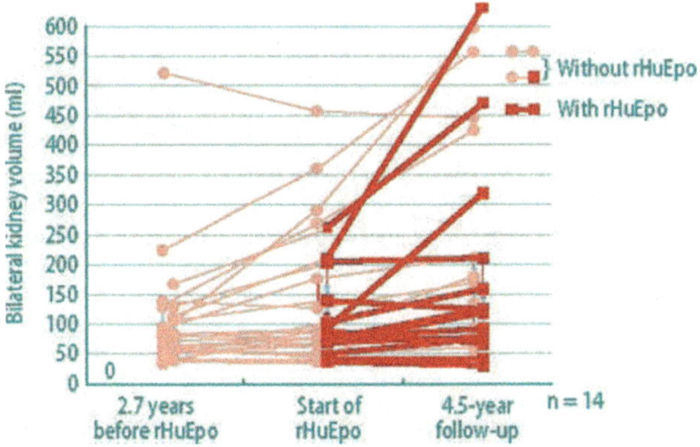

FIG. 22. Changes in kidney volume in male patients with a 5-year history of hemodialysis or longer with and without erythropoietin (rHuEpo) administration

8 Effects of Renal Transplantation

After renal transplantation, ACDK regresses. Following successful renal transplantation, acquired cysts regressed in a few months, and both kidneys markedly decreased in size [44] (Fig. 23). This phenomenon was so surprising that at first I wondered whether I had misread the photographs. Later, I also encountered a case in which the cysts had almost disappeared as early as 4 weeks after transplantation [10] (Fig. 24). The regression of cysts after renal transplantation was also a common phenomenon in other cases (Fig. 25). A recent evaluation also demonstrated that regression starts within 1 month after transplantation, i.e., during the recovery period from acute tubular necrosis (ATN) [45]. The mechanisms of the regression of cysts may be as follows. (1) Most importantly, the serum creatinine level becomes almost normal,

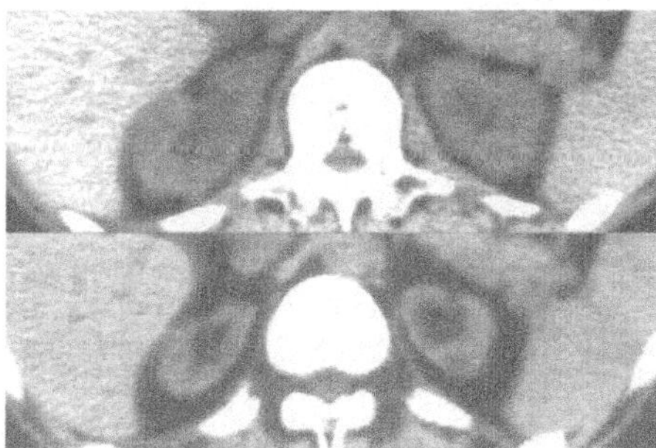

FIG. 23. The first image that indicated the regression of acquired cystic disease of the kidney after successful renal transplantation (Reproduced from [44], with permission from S. Karger AG)

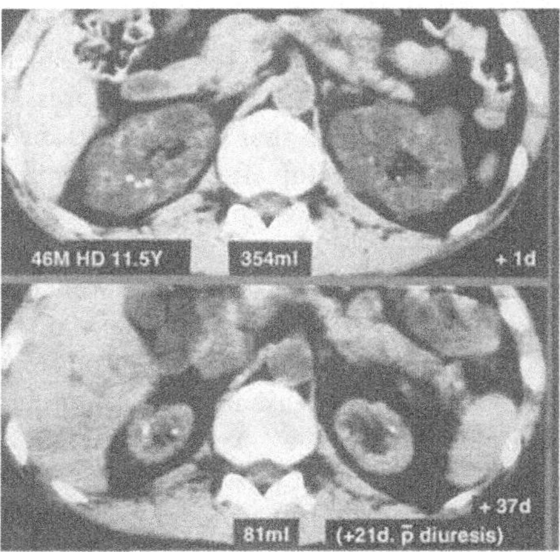

FIG. 24. Regression of acquired cystic disease of the kidney after renal transplantation (Reproduced from [11], with permission from S. Karger AG)

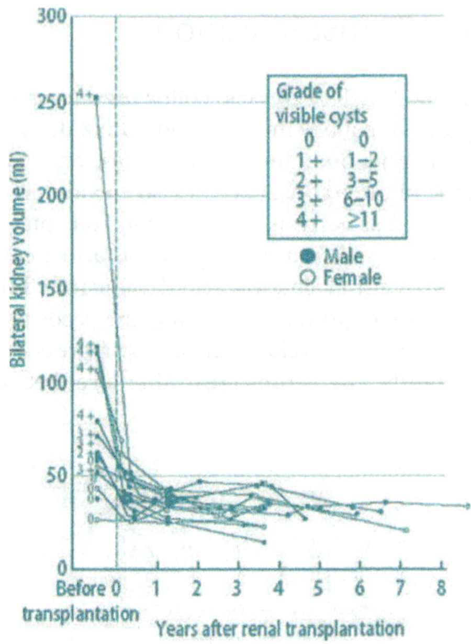

FIG. 25. Changes in kidney volume after renal transplantation. A decrease in kidney volume due to the regression of acquired cysts was observed immediately after transplantation

which will resolve the uremic environment. (2) The blood flow in the native kidney decreases with a decrease in osmotic pressure load. This is caused by a decrease in the urine volume from the native kidney after transplantation of a graft kidney. (3) The cysts are smaller and have more communication with renal tubules and glomeruli in ACDK than in ADPKD [30]. (4) If there are cyst proliferation factors [46], they may not be removed by dialysis, but they may be excreted into the urine by the graft kidney even if its renal function is not adequate. (5) Immunosuppressants induce shrinkage of renal cysts. However, there are no data that support this mechanism, and there is a report that cysts are more likely to develop after renal transplantation if cyclosporin (CsA) is used [47]. Therefore, using my own protocol, I examined the patients with highly functional grafted kidneys from a group who had received renal transplantation using cyclosporin. I observed no difference in parenchymal atrophy or cyst regression of the native kidney after renal transplantation, or in the development of new cysts, whether or not cyclosporin was used [48]. (6) Cells of the cyst wall in ACDK decrease due to apoptosis, causing a decrease in cysts. Eventually, ACDK may transform into the original atrophic kidneys.

Recently, a 20% decrease in the kidney volume was also observed in a patient in whom renal function had just begun to improve, and the graft kidney had excreted only 400 ml/day urine (Fig. 26). I now present some cases of patients in which the cysts disappeared almost completely as early as 2 weeks after transplantation. The first patient (Fig. 27) was a 52-year-old man who had received dialysis for 231 months

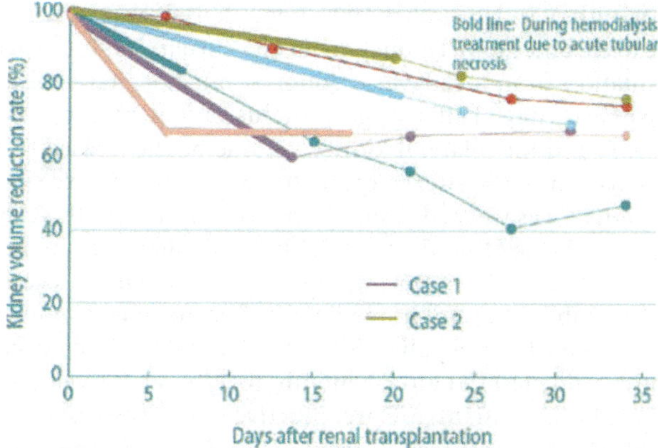

FIG. 26. The rate of decrease in kidney volume during the first month after renal transplantation. The kidney volume began to decrease because of a regression of cysts even when the urine volume was low due to acute tubular necrosis. Case 1 showed an early decrease, and Case 2 showed a slow decrease

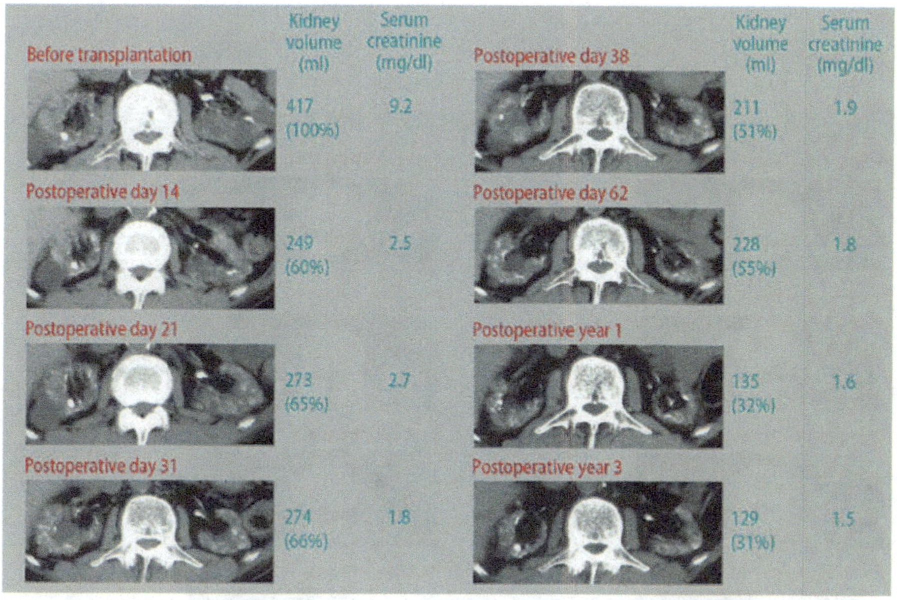

FIG. 27. Regression of acquired renal cysts early after renal transplantation. Regression began even during the period of acute tubular necrosis in a case that showed early regression (Case 1 in Fig. 26)

(19 years and 3 months). In November 1997, hemodialysis was initiated for terminal renal failure due to chronic glomerulonephritis. In February 1997, the patient received a renal transplantation from a cadaveric donor at our hospital, and underwent the first postoperative CT on day 14 after surgery. In this patient, renal cysts were observed on preoperative CT, and the bilateral kidney volume had increased to 417 ml. Urine began to be excreted on day 4 after surgery, the urine volume exceeded 1000 ml on day 12, and the patient was weaned from dialysis on day 14. On this day, the first CT after transplantation showed that the bilateral kidney volume was reduced to 249 ml, or 60% of the preoperative value. During this period, the patient's serum creatinine level decreased from about 9 mg/dl immediately after the operation to about 3 mg/dl (Fig. 27). In the second case, the patient's bilateral kidney volume decreased to 75% of the preoperative value (100%) after 1 month, to 17% after 1 year, and to 13% (or 44 ml) after 3 years. In this patient, the preoperative size of the cysts was smaller than in the first patient, and they occurred in groups (Fig. 28). The regression of cysts after renal transplantation may provide an important clue to an evaluation of the etiology of ACDK.

Thereafter, detailed examinations of cysts in native kidneys after renal transplantation showed that the cysts remained regressed if the renal function was adequate, but that new cysts developed occasionally [49]. These cysts may have been simple renal cysts. However, an exploration for tumors is essential if cysts in the native kidney do not regress [50] or if they enlarge [51] after renal transplantation [52,53].

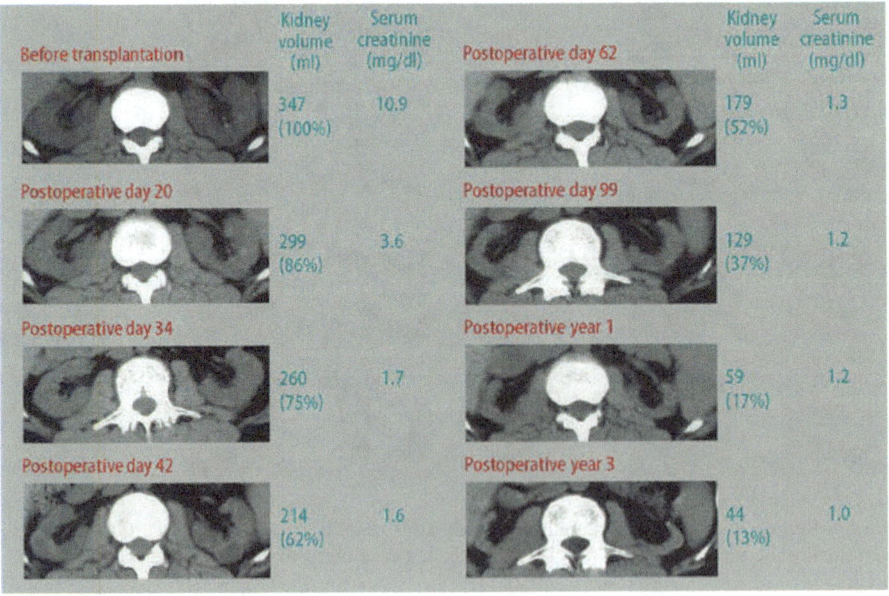

FIG. 28. Regression of acquired renal cysts early after renal transplantation. A case that showed slow regression (Case 2 in Fig. 26)

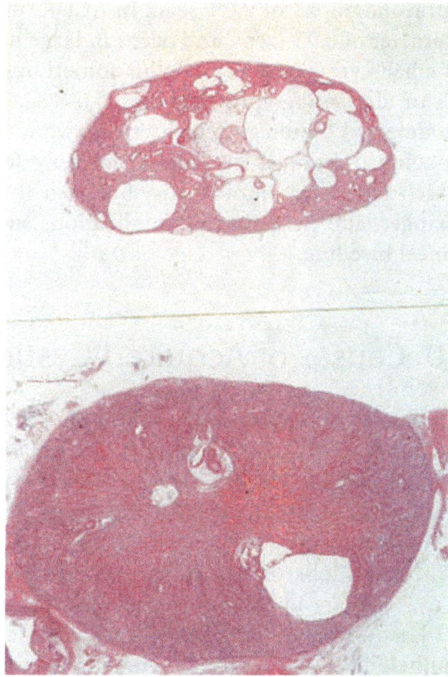

FIG. 29. Many cysts appeared in the native kidney (*above*) with the decline in the function of the graft kidney. Since the period of chronic renal failure was short (*below*), fewer cysts developed in the graft kidney than in the native kidney (Reproduced from [54], with permission from Elsevier Inc.)

TABLE 2. Clinical characteristics of acquired cysts in acquired cystic disease of the kidney

1. High incidence of renal cell carcinoma
2. Relationship to the duration of chronic renal failure and hemodialysis
3. Male preponderance
4. No relationship to dialysis modality
5. No relationship to dialysis membrane
6. Regression of acquired cysts after renal transplantation

Naturally, if the function of the graft kidney is reduced, cysts again increase in the native kidney. A small number of cysts also appear in the graft kidney if reduced function persists [54] (Fig. 29).

The clinical characteristics of acquired cysts in ACDK are summarized in Table 2.

9 Diagnosis of Acquired Cystic Disease of the Kidney

Acquired cystic disease of the kidney can be diagnosed if a total of three to five cysts are found in one kidney (or three to five cysts in both kidneys combined according to some authors) on an imaging study [11]. The imaging technique may be either ultrasonography or a CT scan. In ACDK, the cysts are characteristically small, with a diameter of 0.02–2 cm, and occur in large numbers. In cross sections, a large number of small cysts are observed, but sometimes only one cyst on the top can be seen by CT or ultrasonography (see Fig. 11). Cysts 0.5 cm or greater in diameter can usually be detected by imaging techniques, while smaller cysts are undetectable. However, imaging techniques are useful not only for the diagnosis of renal cell carcinoma, which is rarely symptomatic, but also for an evaluation of the severity of cystic changes, and the risks of complications such as renal cell carcinoma and retroperitoneal bleeding.

10 Causes of Acquired Cystic Disease of the Kidney

Why do cysts develop and grow in the kidneys in end-stage renal failure or after the initiation of dialysis? At present, the causes or pathogenic mechanism of such cysts remain unclear. During the past 26 years, many hypotheses have been proposed, as shown in Table 3, including proliferation of the tubular epithelium due to uremic metabolites and growth factors, ischemia, factors related to hemodialysis such as plasticizers, obstruction of the renal tubules by oxalate crystals, β_2-microglobulins, etc., hormone imbalance, trace elements such as vanadium, and regional acidosis [10]. However, all these hypotheses, with the exception of proliferation of the tubular epithelium due to uremic metabolites and growth factors, are currently considered to be unlikely.

Since cysts enlarge during long-term dialysis whether it is hemodialysis or CAPD, and since they regress after successful renal transplantation [44], I speculated that proliferation of the tubular epithelium due to uremic metabolites and growth factors is involved in the mechanism of cyst formation (Table 3), and that these uremic metabolites and growth factors are mainly active in males. However, these factors remain to be identified.

It is also of interest that the cyst fluid of ACDK showed a different pattern compared with the cyst fluid of ADPKD or of simple renal cysts on examination using a surface-enhanced laser desorption/ionization time-of-flight mass spectrometer (SELDI-TOF-MS) and ProteinChips. These findings are being analyzed (Fig. 30).

TABLE 3. Hypotheses of the pathogenic mechanisms of acquired cystic disease of the kidney

1. Epithelial hyperplasia theory due to:
   Uremic metabolites and/or growth factors due to the loss of functioning nephrons
   Ischemia
   A dialysis-related substance (plasticizer, etc)
2. Tubular obstruction theory due to:
   Oxalate crystals, β_2-microglobulin, etc
3. Other theory (trace element-vanadium, regional acidosis)

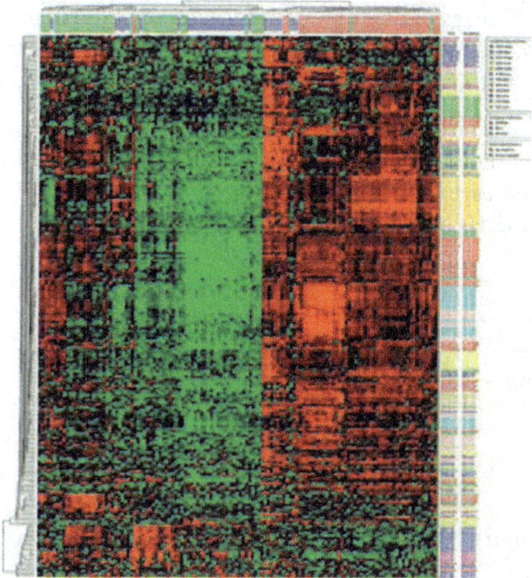

FIG. 30. A heat-map showing the results of proteome analysis of cyst fluid by SELDI-TOF-MS. Proteins in the cyst fluid of acquired renal cysts are classified into different clusters. The clusters indicate, from left to right, acquired cystic disease of the kidney without renal cell carcinoma, acquired cystic disease of the kidney with renal cell carcinoma, and autosomal dominant polycystic kidney disease. Proteins in some cysts of acquired cystic disease of the kidney with renal cell carcinoma revealed clusters which were similar to those of autosomal dominant polycystic kidney disease

11 Twenty-Year Follow-up of Acquired Cystic Disease of the Kidney

We followed up 96 patients who had undergone renal function replacement therapy for chronic glomerulonephritis since 1979 [13]. During this period, 44 died, 36 required hemodialysis (19 males and 17 females) and could be followed up for 20 years, and 7 were managed for 20 years by renal transplantation alone. During this period, renal cell carcinoma occurred in 6 patients and 4 of these died, but the deaths were not due to the renal cell carcinoma. Table 4 shows the causes of death in the 44 patients. Enlargement of the kidneys was observed more frequently in male patients than in female patients. Figure 31 shows the severity of cystic changes. After 20 years, advanced grade 4 cystic changes were observed in many male patients. When the male patients were divided into those aged less than 40 years and those aged 40 years and above, and the percentages of those who showed a 4-fold or greater enlargement of the kidneys were compared, the kidneys were enlarged due to cysts more often in those aged less than 40 years. In other words, cysts among male patients were found to be more likely to develop in relatively young subjects.

Figure 32 shows the CT scans for this study. Images of a 47-year-old man who had undergone hemodialysis for 1 year and 7 months are shown on the left. His kidney

TABLE 4. Causes of death in patients who died during a 20-year follow-up of acquired cystic disease of the kidney (Reproduced from [13], with permission from Dustri-Verlag Dr. Karl Feistle)

Causes of death in 44 patients		
Myocardial infarction	8 (+RCC)	(18.2%)
Congestive heart failure	7	(15.9%)
Cerebrovascular accident	7 (+RCC)	(15.9%)
Malignancy	7	(15.9%)
Stomach	1 (+RCC)	
Rectum	1	
Pancreas	1	
Myeloma	1	
Uterus	2 (+RCC)	
Breast	1	
Infection	5	(11.4%)
Cachexia	2	(4.5%)
Hepatic failure	2	(4.5%)
Accident	2	(4.5%)
Ileus	2	(4.5%)
Retroperitoneal bleeding	1	(2.3%)
Respiratory failure	1	(2.3%)

RCC, renal cell carcinoma

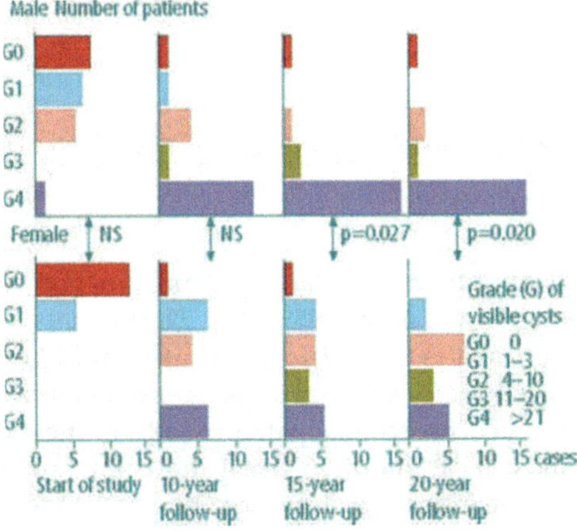

FIG. 31. A 20-year follow-up of acquired cystic disease of the kidney. The graphs show the frequencies of the grades of cysts during the follow-up. Severe grade-4 cystic changes were observed in many of the male patients after 20 years (Reproduced from [13], with permission from Dustri-Verlag Dr. Karl Feistle)

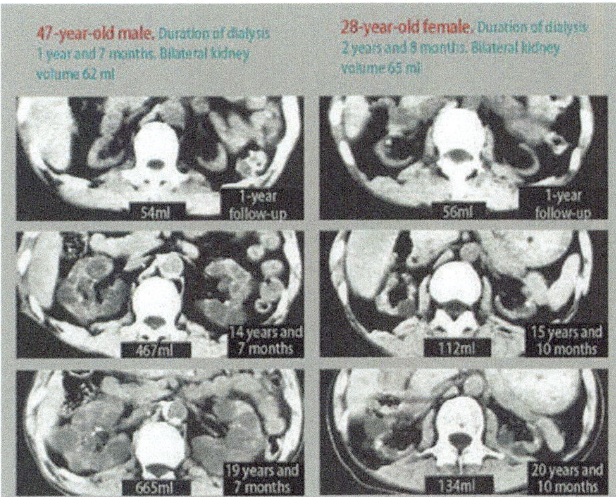

Fig. 32. A 20-year follow-up of acquired cystic disease of the kidney. Images of a male and a female patient during the follow-up. Sex differences are evident (Reproduced from [13], with permission from Dustri-Verlag Dr. Karl Feistle)

volume, which was originally 62 ml, decreased slightly to 54 ml after 1 year, but increased markedly to 467 ml after 15 years, and to 665 ml after 20 years, but with increases in the number of cysts. Images of a 28-year-old woman who had undergone dialysis for 2 years and 8 months are shown on the right. Very few cysts developed during the 20-year follow-up period, and her kidney volume, which was originally 65 ml, was 56 ml, 112 ml, and 134 ml after 1 year, 15 years, and 20 years, respectively, which were much smaller increases. To summarize the results of our 20-year follow-up, cystic changes in the kidney were more notable in male patients, and the kidney volume showed marked increases, particularly in young male patients. Although renal cell carcinoma was detected in six patients during this period, they all died of unrelated reasons.

Chapter 3
Renal Cell Carcinomas in Dialysis Patients

1 The Two Types of Renal Cell Carcinoma in Dialysis Patients

Two types of renal cell carcinoma (RCC) are found in dialysis patients, i.e., those that complicate and those that do not complicate acquired cystic disease of the kidney (ACDK). The type that complicates ACDK accounts for 81% of all renal cell carcinomas, and is observed more frequently in male patients, younger patients, and patients who have been managed longer by dialysis than the type which does not complicate this disease [55]. Histologically, the type of renal cell carcinoma that complicates ACDK is most often papillary renal cell carcinoma, which is closely related to cysts. On the other hand, the type of renal cell carcinoma that does not complicate ACDK is frequently observed in elderly patients, its occurrence is unrelated to the duration of dialysis therapy, and the percentage of clear cell carcinomas is high.

2 Histology

When acquired cystic disease of the kidney (ACDK) is complicated by renal cell carcinoma, the kidney size varies with the duration of dialysis and the sex of the patient, and may become indistinguishable from that of kidneys with autosomal dominant polycystic kidney disease (ADPKD) [23].

Figure 33 shows a kidney of a 64-year-old man who had received hemodialysis for 13 years. Multiple cysts were observed in the bilateral kidneys, and a mass 4.5 cm in diameter was noted in the lower pole of the right kidney. When the resected kidney was cut along the same planes as the CT slices (Fig. 34), renal cell carcinomas (represented as areas with red diagonal lines), cysts with monolayer epithelium (surrounded by a black line), multilayered so-called atypical cysts (surrounded by a red or blue line), and solid adenomas (represented as areas of solid color) were distributed in a multicentric pattern. Such simultaneous presence of cysts, atypical cysts, solid adenomas, and renal cell carcinomas in the same kidney, their multicentric occurrence, and the presence of precancerous lesions are histological characteristics of ACDK [1,11]. Renal cell carcinoma is bilateral in 9%–15% of patients [56–58].

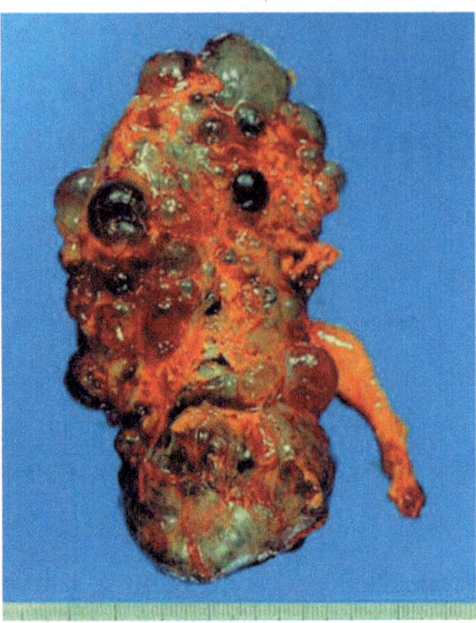

FIG. 33. A macroscopic image of acquired cystic disease of the kidney in a 64-year-old man with a 13-year history of hemodialysis. A renal cell carcinoma can be seen in the lower pole

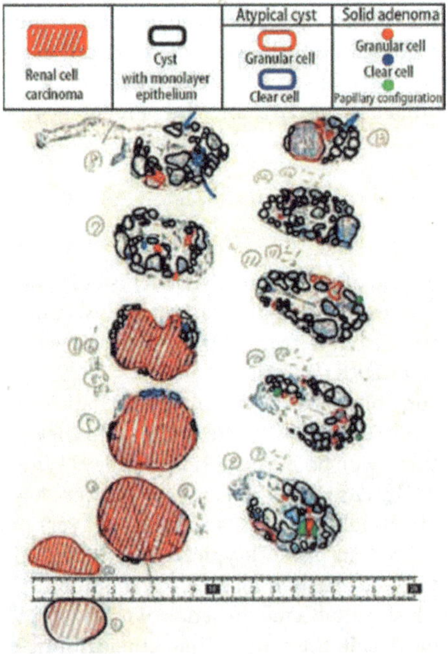

FIG. 34. Cross-sectional pathology of the resected kidney shown in FIG. 33. Cysts, atypical cysts, solid adenoma, and renal cell carcinoma were seen in the same kidney

As shown in Fig. 35, microscopic examination showed that this patient had (a) proximal tubules with epithelial hyperplasia, (b) cysts with monolayer epithelium, (c) atypical cysts with multilayered epithelium, (d) adenoma, and (e) papillary renal cell carcinoma.

Acquired cystic disease of the kidney characteristically shows precancerous lesions such as atypical cysts and adenomas. The presence of the brush border (microvilli) in the cyst epithelium and the composition of the cyst fluid suggest a proximal tubular origin for the cysts (both cysts with monolayer epithelium and atypical cysts). On examination of their proliferative ability using vimentin, EGF receptor, and c-erb B2, 73% of atypical cysts were positive for vimentin, 95% were positive for EGF receptor [59], and 100% were positive for c-erb B2 [59,60]. However, only 9.7% of the samples

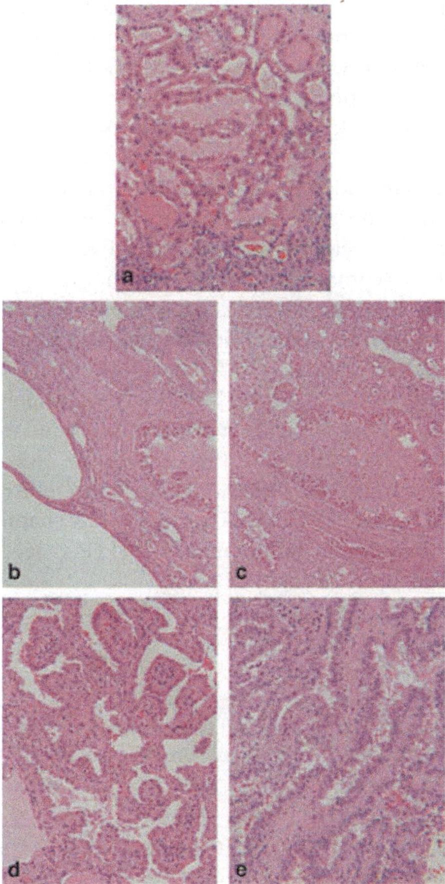

FIG. 35. Microscopic images. **a** Hyperplastic proximal tubules. **b** Cyst with monolayer epithelium. **c** Atypical cyst with multilayer epithelium. **d** Adenoma. **e** Papillary renal cell carcinoma

of the cyst walls with monolayer epithelium were positive for c-erb B2. These findings indicate that cyst epithelial cells of patients with ACDK have high proliferative ability.

Concerning the proliferative ability of renal cell carcinomas of dialysis patients, the doubling time varied widely between those which grew slowly and those which grew rapidly. According to Takebayashi et al. [61], the doubling time of tumors varied from 0.08 to 23.31 years (5.09 ± 6.99 years), and the rate of increase in cyst volume varied from 0.07 to 17.34 cm^3/year (4.14 ± 5.66 cm^3/year).

Dunnill et al. [1] classified the renal tumors of dialysis patients as papillary, tubular, or solid tumors, and Ishikawa and Kovacs [62] showed that a higher percentage of papillary renal cell carcinomas occurred in dialysis patients than in patients who had not undergone dialysis (Table 5). This result appears reasonable because of the relationship between papillary renal cell carcinoma and cysts. According to a recent questionnaire [63] of patients in whom renal cell carcinoma was recorded, 55% were clear cell carcinomas and 18% were papillary renal cell carcinomas in dialysis patients, but 83% were clear cell carcinomas and 5% were papillary renal cell carcinomas in nondialysis patients. In addition, it was shown that while clear cell carcinoma develops at any time after the initiation of dialysis, papillary renal cell carcinoma increases as dialysis is continued over a longer period. Both tumors may occur in the same kidney.

Other histological types include oncocytoma [64,65], chromophobe renal cell carcinoma, Bellini duct tumor, and erythropoietin-producing tumor [66]. Among some rare histological types, one foreign patient [67] and five Japanese patients [68–71] (including Case 33) with sarcomatoid renal cell carcinoma (spindle cell carcinoma) with a poor outcome [50], and cystic renal cell carcinoma with a good outcome [72], have been reported. Transitional cell carcinoma has also been observed, although rarely, as well as renal cell carcinoma [73,74].

As mentioned, in a survey in 2004 [63] of the histological types of a total of 1049 cases of renal cell carcinoma, based on the General Rule for Clinical and Pathological Studies on Renal Cell Carcinoma in 1999, there were 565 clear cell carcinomas (53.9%), 197 granular cell carcinomas (18.8%), 12 chromophobe renal cell carcinomas (1.1%), 68 cyst-associated renal cell carcinomas (6.5%), 180 papillary renal cell carcinomas (17.2%), and 27 spindle cell carcinomas (2.6%) (Fig. 36).

TABLE 5. Comparison of the histology of renal cell carcinoma in the general population and in hemodialysis patients (Reproduced from [62], with permission from Blackwell Publishing)

	General population	Hemodialysis patients
Nonpapillary RCC	73* (88.0%)	22* (51.2%)
Papillary renal cell tumor	4* (4.8%)	21* (48.8%)
Chromophobe RCC	6 (7.2%)	0
Number of cases	83	43

*χ^2 = 31.9, p < 0.001. RCC, renal cell carcinoma

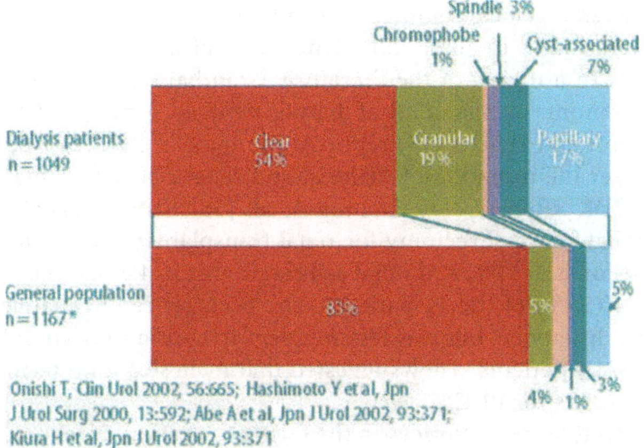

Fig. 36. Comparison of the histological characteristics of renal cell carcinomas between dialysis patients and the general population. In dialysis patients, clear cell carcinoma is less frequent, and granular cell carcinoma and papillary renal cell carcinoma are more frequent, than in the general population. Papillary renal cell carcinoma is particularly frequent in renal cell carcinoma related to acquired cystic disease of the kidney

TABLE 6. Prevalence of acquired cystic disease of the kidney, renal tumors, and renal cell carcinoma as reported in the literature

Total cases from 25 references examined (CT, US, autopsy)	Cysts (ACDK)	Renal tumor	RCC
1103 Cases	520 Cases (47.1%)	53 Cases (4.8%)	17 Cases (1.5%)

CT, computed tomography

3 Prevalence

In relation to the prevalence of renal cell carcinoma observed in 1103 dialysis patients, as reported in the literature (including imaging and pathological diagnoses), cysts were observed in 47.1%, renal tumors in 4.8%, and renal cell carcinomas in 1.5% [14] (Table 6).

According to the results of my 10-year follow-up data, the annual incidence of renal cell carcinoma was 0.4% [34]. Based on a questionnaire survey in 2004 it was 0.2%, and in a 20-year follow-up study it was 0.3%. This means that the first screening of 100 patients at a dialysis center reveals renal cell carcinoma in 1–2 dialysis patients, and further screenings of the same group reveal the disease in 1 patient every 2.5 years thereafter.

Acquired renal cysts are observed in about 50% of dialysis patients, and since the prevalence of renal cell carcinoma is 1.5%, about 3% of the patients with ACDK are expected to have renal cell carcinoma. According to the data of Hughson et al. [75], atypical cysts were found in 30%, and adenoma in 14%, of the kidneys of patients receiving dialysis. In a review of the literature, Grantham and Levine [76] reported that renal cell carcinoma occurs in 7% of dialysis patients. Among recent pathological evaluations, Segerer and Meister [77] reported adenoma in 10%–20% of patients with ACDK 3 years after the initiation of dialysis, and renal cell carcinoma in 3%–6% of patients with ACDK after 5 years. Denton et al. [56] histologically examined 260 patients after unilateral nephrectomy for renal transplantation, and found acquired cysts in 33%, adenoma in 14%, and renal cell carcinoma in 4.2%; renal cell carcinoma was bilateral in 4 (36%) of the 11 patients. The occurrence of renal cell carcinoma showed no racial difference, but was less frequent in continuous ambulatory perito-neal dialysis (CAPD) patients. They suggested that male sex, long-term dialysis, and aging were risk factors for RCC.

We carried out a total of 12 surveys in the form of questionnaires concerning renal cell carcinoma in dialysis patients every 2 years from 1982 to 2004 [55,57,63,78–86]. Based on the results of the surveys in 1996–2004, the annual incidence of renal cell carcinoma was found to be 146–191 per 100000 patients (0.146%–0.191% of all patients). However, it was 88–112 per 100000 (0.088%–0.112%) in patients with a history of less than 10 years dialysis, but it was 344–438 per 100000 (0.344%–0.438%) in those who had undergone dialysis for 10 years or longer. These figures show that the incidence of renal cell carcinoma increases with the duration of dialysis, and that this increase is about four times greater in those with a 10-year history of dialysis or longer compared with those with a history of less than 10 years (Fig. 37).

We also compared the prevalence of renal cell carcinoma in dialysis patients with that in the general population, using sex- and age-matched subjects based on the results of our questionnaires, i.e., we calculated the standardized incidence ratio (SIR) [63]. According to the results from 2004, the SIR was 14.8 (95% CI, 13.1–16.7) in all patients, 14.3 (95% CI, 12.4–16.7) in males, and 17.1 (95% CI, 12.9–23.2) in females (Fig. 38). The incidence of renal cell carcinoma was 9–18 times higher in male patients and 8–17 times higher in female patients than in the general population, and 0.8–2.0

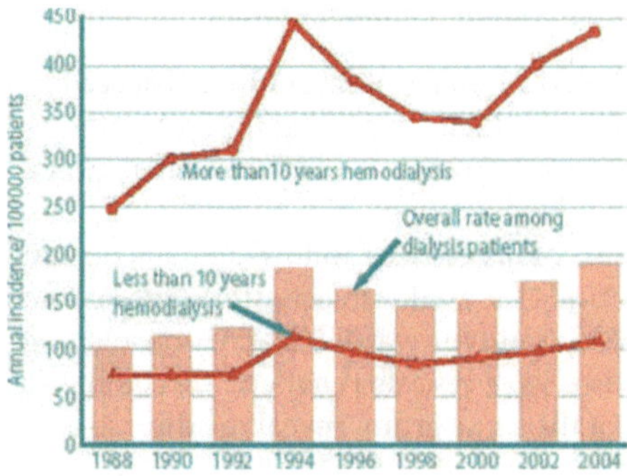

FIG. 37. Annual incidence of renal cell carcinoma per 100000 dialysis patients, and the duration of dialysis (Reproduced from [63], with permission)

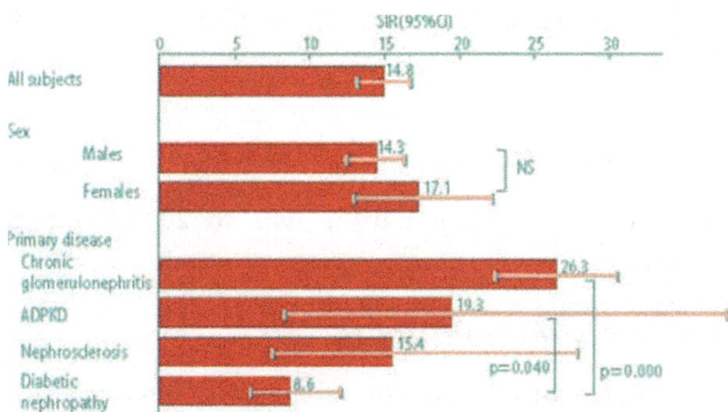

FIG. 38. Standardized incidence ratio (SIR) of renal cell carcinoma in dialysis patients and their 95% confidence intervals

TABLE 7. Comparison of the standardized incidence ratio (SIR) of renal cell carcinoma in male and female hemodialysis patients in each questionnaire (Reproduced from [63], with permission)

Questionnaire year	Males	Females	Male/Female
1990	16.5	8.3	2.0
1992	16.9	12.1	1.4
1994	18.2	15.0	1.2
1996	14.7	11.7	1.3
1998	9.7	9.3	1.0
2000	8.9	9.1	1.0
2002	13.1	15.2	0.9
2004	14.3	17.1	0.8

times higher in male patients than in female patients (Table 7). In patients aged less than 40 years, in particular, the incidence was 54–143 times higher in male patients and 284–412 times higher in female patients. As the survey was repeated over time, the incidence in female patients increased [63], and the male predominance gradually became less conspicuous.

In 2003, Stewart et al. [87] analyzed the cases reported in a registry covering three continents, and reported that the incidence of renal cell carcinoma was 2053 (United States Renal Data System: USRDS 1303; European Dialysis and Transplantation Association: EDTA 680; Australia/New Zealand: A/NZ 70) per 2 045 035 patient-years (0.100%). The SIR of renal cell carcinoma (International Classification of Disease: ICD-9 189, renal cell carcinoma and tumors of the urinary system except bladder cancer) was high at 3.6 in all patients, was higher in younger patients, and was higher in female patients (4.6) than in male patients (3.2). These tendencies were observed regardless of the primary disease (Fig. 38). Thus, the occurrence of renal cell carcinoma is dependent on the duration of dialysis rather than on the primary disease or dialysis modality, and increases as the duration of dialysis increases (SIR = 3.2 at 1 year, 3.7 at 3–5 years, and 6.8 at 10 years or longer).

4 Results of Surveys Concerning Renal Cell Carcinoma in Dialysis Patients

4.1 Results in 1982–2004

The results of the surveys performed from 1982 to 2004 are presented below [55,57,63,78–86,88,89].

4.2 Number of Registered Patients

We were able to collect data for 2873 dialysis patients with renal cell carcinoma (Table 8). When the annual rate of increase was compared between renal cell carcinoma patients and dialysis patients, it was found to be slightly higher in renal cell carcinoma patients (Fig. 39).

4.3 Sex Differences

We know that acquired renal cysts are observed more frequently in male patients, and in these surveys of dialysis patients, renal cell carcinoma was observed in 2293 males (80%), 574 females (20%), and 6 patients of unknown gender. The prevalence was four times higher in male patients than in female patients. However, Stewart

TABLE 8. Number of dialysis patients with renal cell carcinoma as collected by questionnaire surveys (Reproduced from [63], with permission)

	1982	1984	1986	1988	1990	1992	1994	1996	1998	2000	2002	2004	Total
Males	25	31	40	91	112	150	216	222	285	320	381	420	2293 (80.0%)
Females	9	6	8	24	18	34	57	55	68	79	104	112	574 (20.0%)
Unknown											4	2	6
Total	34	37	48	115	130	184	273	277	353	399	489	534	2873

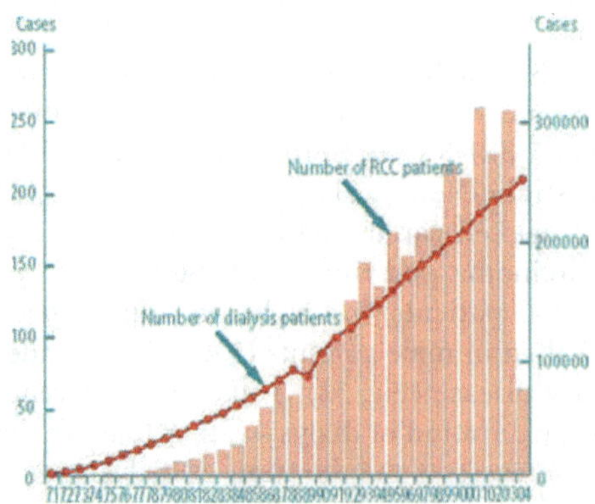

FIG. 39. Annual changes in the numbers of renal cell carcinoma patients and dialysis patients

et al. [87] reported that the SIR was slightly higher in female patients than in male patients, and our data were similar (SIR 14.3 in males, 17.1 in females).

4.4 Age

The mean age of patients with renal cell carcinoma is lower (55.5 ± 11.5 years) than that of the general population, and many patients with renal cell carcinoma were in their 30s or 40s (Fig. 40). The mean age of patients with renal cell carcinoma also increased at every survey. It was 47.9 years in 1982 (51.9 years at the end of 1983, 48.3 years at the initiation of dialysis), but was 58.9 ± 10.9 years in 2004, i.e., it had increased by 11 years during the 20 years of the surveys (Table 9). The mean age of all dialysis patients also increased by 15.1 years from 47.1 years during the same period (Fig. 41). The mean ages of both the renal cell carcinoma patients and all the

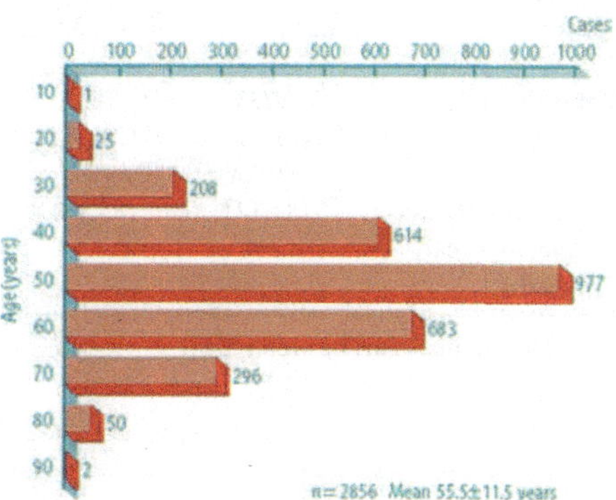

FIG. 40. Age distribution of renal cell carcinoma patients

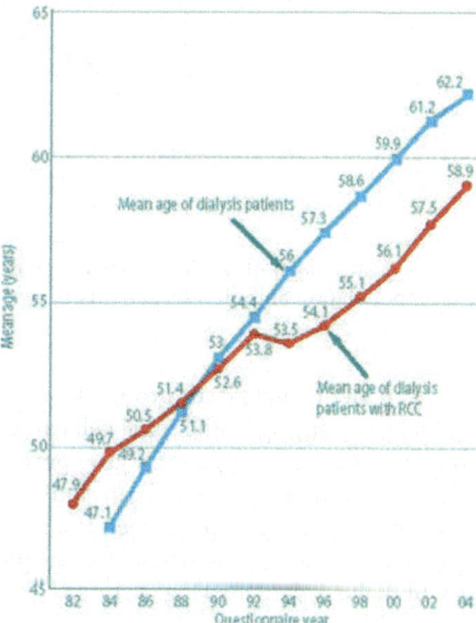

FIG 41 Annual changes in the mean age of dialysis patients with and without renal cell carcinoma

TABLE 9. Summary of the results of surveys from 1982 to 2004 (Reproduced from [63], with permission)

	1982a	1984	1986	1988	1990	1992
Number of RCC patients	34	37	48	115	130	184
Males	25	31	40	91	112	150 (81.5%)
Females	9	6	8	24	18	34 (18.5%)
Male:Female	2.8:1	5.2:1	5.0:1	3.8:1	6.2:1	4.4:1
Mean age (years)	47.9±15.6b	49.7±11.1	50.5±10.0	51.4±11.7	52.6±10.9	53.8±11.8 (183)
Mean duration of dialysis (months)	49.4 ± 32.8	73.6 ± 46.3	83.9 ± 45.2	94.6 ± 54.5	106.1 ± 61.2	111.0 ± 64.3 (183)
Presence of acquired cysts (%)	23/32 (71.9)	20/32 (62.5)	39/46 (84.8)	92/115 (80.0)	102/124 (82.3)	142/179 (79.3)
Tumor size (cm)	4.25±3.21	4.90±3.99	5.39±3.78	4.58±3.44	4.22±2.53	4.70±3.20 (166)
Metastasis (%)	7/33 (21.2)	8/33 (24.2)	10/48 (20.8)	17/106 (16.0)	19/126 (15.1)	29/182 (15.9)
Total number of dialysis patients in Japan (year, month)	42 223 (81.12)	53 017 (83.12)	66 310 (85.12)	80 553 (87.12)	88 534 (88.12)	116 303 (90.12)

a, Questionnaire year; b, Mean ± SD

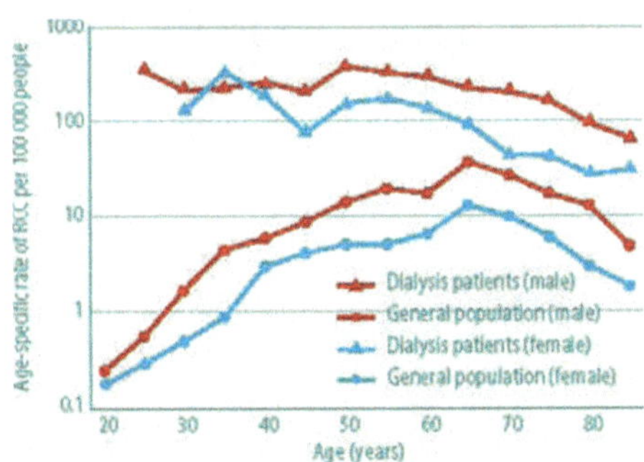

FIG. 42. Comparison of the incidence of renal cell carcinoma per 100 000 people between the general population and dialysis patients according to sex and age

dialysis patients increased, probably because the age at the initiation of dialysis was gradually increasing, while renal cell carcinoma occurred more frequently in patients who had received dialysis for a long period from a relatively young age, and because renal cell carcinoma occurred at relatively young ages in dialysis patients.

When the relationship between the incidence of renal cell carcinoma and age was evaluated separately in male and female patients, the incidence was higher at younger ages in dialysis patients (Fig. 42).

1994	1996	1998	2000	2002	2004	Total
273	277	353	399	489	534	2873
216	222	285	320	381	420	2293
(79.1%)	(80.1%)	(80.7%)	(80.2%)	(78.6%)	(78.9%)	(80.0%)
57	55	68	79	104	112	574
(20.9%)	(19.9%)	(19.3%)	(19.8%)	(21.4%)	(21.1%)	(20.0%)
3.8:1	4.0:1	4.2:1	4.1:1	3.7:1	3.8:1	4.0:1
53.5±11.3	54.1±11.7	55.1±11.3	56.1±10.7	57.5±11.4	58.9±10.9	55.5±11.5
(272)	(276)	(348)	(397)	(484)	(533)	(2856)
118.2 ± 71.0	125.8 ± 79.5	131.5 ± 87.9	132.8 ± 85.8	136.9 ± 95.2	145.7 ± 95.0	126.9 ± 84.9
(271)	(276)	(345)	(392)	(464)	(529)	(2831)
224/271	222/271	293/345	304/380	384/476	422/518	2267/2789
(82.7)	(81.9)	(84.9)	(80.0)	(80.7)	(81.5)	(81.3)
4.00±2.70	3.98±2.81	3.96±2.37	3.96±2.92	3.77±2.40	3.53±2.01	3.97±2.67
(242)	(260)	(323)	(360)	(464)	(505)	(2653)
35/269	45/273	56/341	57/379	72/473	73/524	428/2787
(13.0)	(16.5)	(16.4)	(15.0)	(15.2)	(13.9)	(15.4)
123 000	143 709	167 192	185 322	206 134	229 538	
(92.12)	(94.12)	(96.12)	(98.12)	(00.12)	(02.12)	

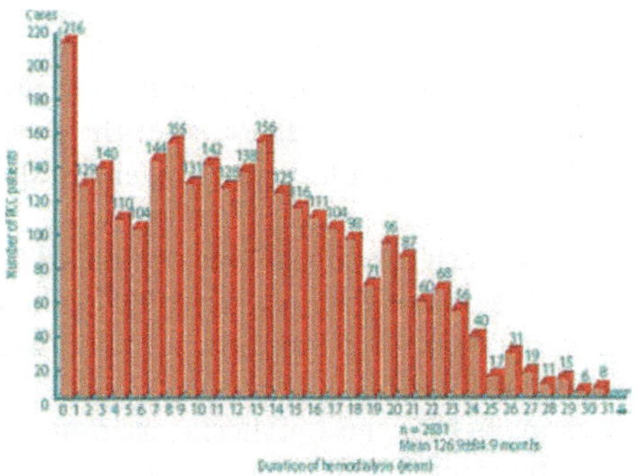

FIG. 43. Duration of dialysis and number of renal cell carcinoma patients

4.5 Duration of Dialysis

The mean duration of dialysis in renal cell carcinoma patients was 126.9 ± 84.9 months (10.6 years) (Fig. 43). Renal cell carcinoma occurred more frequently within 1 year or between 5 and 15 years after the initiation of dialysis. The incidence of renal cell carcinoma increased with the duration of dialysis (Fig. 44). According to the results of the survey in 2004, the duration of dialysis was 10 years or longer in 55.6% of the 534 renal cell carcinoma patients, and 20 years or longer in 18.1% [60]. In other

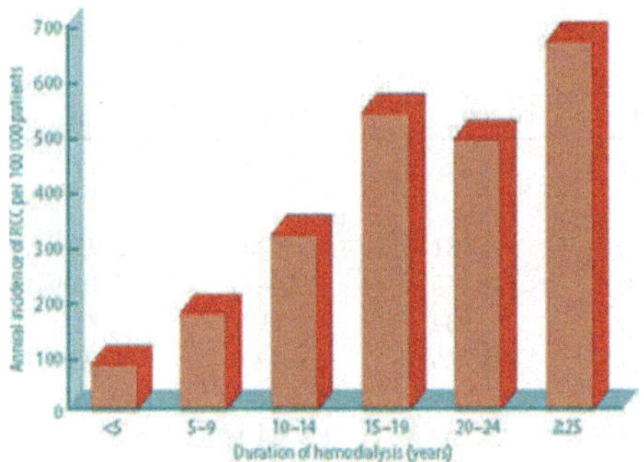

FIG. 44. Comparison of the annual incidence of renal cell carcinoma per 100 000 dialysis patients according to the duration of dialysis

TABLE 10. Comparison of renal cell carcinomas with and without acquired cystic disease of the kidney

	With ACDK	Without ACDK	
n	2267 (81.3%)	522 (18.7%)	
Males	1857 (82.1%)	370 (70.9%)	p = 0.000
Females	405 (17.9%)	152 (29.1%)	
Age (years)	54.7 ± 11.2	58.8 ± 12.1	p = 0.000
Duration of dialysis (months)	142.2 ± 81.8	63.0 ± 66.9	p = 0.000
Tumor size (cm)	3.9 ± 2.6	4.1 ± 2.8	NS
Metastasis	327/2220 (14.7%)	77/513 (15.0%)	NS
Outcome (Cancer death)	169/2250 (7.5%)	42/520 (8.1%)	NS

words, the duration of dialysis was 10 years or longer in about half the dialysis patients with renal cell carcinoma. When the results of the surveys were compared, the number of renal cell carcinoma patients with a longer duration of dialysis gradually increased (Table 9).

When the occurrence of renal cell carcinoma was compared between patients with and without acquired cystic disease of the kidney (ACDK), the patients with ACDK complicated by renal cell carcinoma were more often males, were younger, and had a longer duration of dialysis (Table 10).

When a comparison was made between renal cell carcinoma patients with a duration of dialysis of less than 10 years and those with a duration of dialysis of 20 years or longer, those with a longer duration of dialysis were younger, were more often males, more often had acquired cysts, more often had papillary renal cell carcinoma, more often had metastases, and more often died as a result of the renal cell carcinoma [90] (Table 11).

4.6 Aids to Diagnosis

Aids to a diagnosis of renal cell carcinoma were obtained by screening using imaging techniques such as ultrasonography and CT scan in 90% of patients (Fig. 45). Only 7.6% were found to be symptomatic, and therefore screening was shown to be useful.

TABLE 11. Comparison of the prevalence of renal cell carcinoma in patients with a history of dialysis of 10 years or less and those with a history of dialysis of 20 years or longer (Reproduced from [90], with permission from S. Karger AG)

	Less than 10 years	More than 20 years	p value
n	215	84	
Age (years)	59.8 ± 13.1	55.0 ± 7.1	0.001
Males	74.3% (159/214)	90.1% (73/81)	0.003
Presence of acquired cysts	62.5% (130/208)	96.3% (79/82)	0.000
Tumor size (cm)	3.7 ± 2.3	4.3 ± 2.4	0.036
Papillary RCC	8.1% (13/161)	17.5% (10/57)	0.046
Metastasis	10.6% (22/208)	31.3% (25/80)	0.000
Cancer death	3.7% (8/214)	13.1% (11/84)	0.003
Duration of dialysis (months)	49.0 ± 34.2	283.5 ± 32.7	0.000

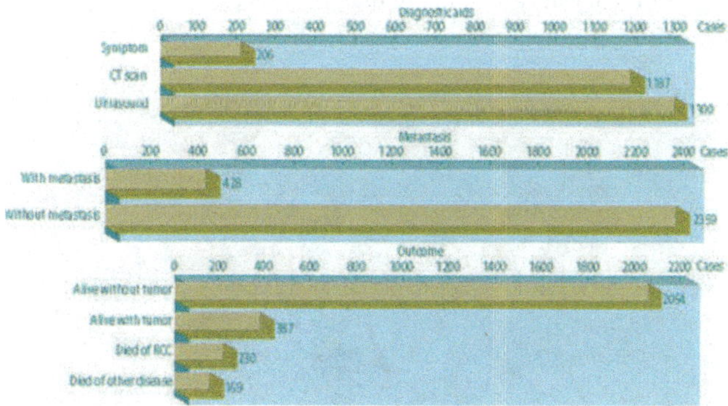

FIG. 45. Diagnostic aids for renal cell carcinoma, metastasis, and outcomes in dialysis patients

4.7 Symptoms

In symptomatic patients (Fig. 46), as expected, the most frequent symptom was gross hematuria (146 cases), and symptoms due to metastasis (20 cases), fever (13), and abdominal/loin pain (10) were also observed. It is noteworthy that an increase in the hematocrit or erythrocytosis led to the detection of renal cell carcinoma in 9 patients (Fig. 46).

4.8 Metastasis

Metastasis occurred in 428 (15.4%) of 2787 cases (Table 9).

4.9 Outcome

The outcome after a mean follow-up period of 1 year (Fig. 45) was 2054 alive without tumor (72%), 387 alive with tumor (14.5%), 230 dead due to renal cell carcinoma (8%), and 169 dead due to other diseases (6%).

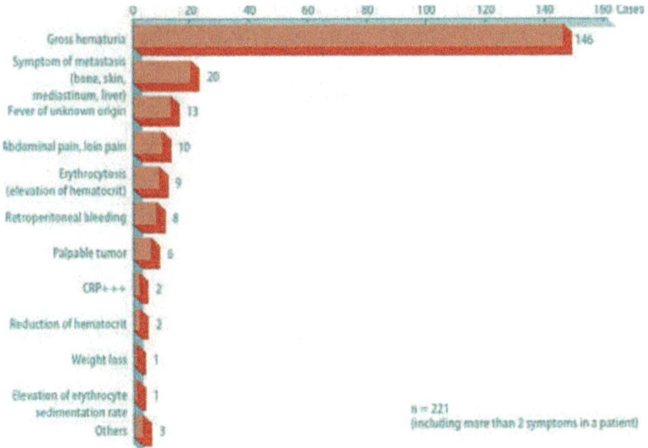

FIG. 46. Symptoms of renal cell carcinoma in dialysis patients

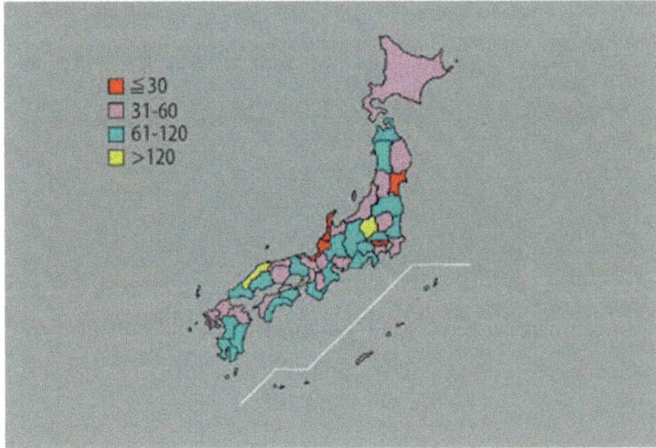

FIG. 47. Comparison of the prevalence of renal cell carcinoma in chronic dialysis patients among prefectures. The prevalence is shown as the number of dialysis patients without renal cell carcinoma for every patient with renal cell carcinoma. The disease is more prevalent when the number is smaller

4.10 Detection Rates in Different Prefectures

The detection rate varied considerably among prefectures. These differences are believed to be caused by the level of interest of the attending physicians in renal cell carcinoma of dialysis patients, and whether or not they performed screening, rather than by regional differences in the incidence of the disease. The detection rate of renal cell carcinoma patients per unit number of dialysis patients was high in Miyagi, Tokyo, Ishikawa, and Fukui prefectures (Fig. 47).

4.11 Size of Renal Cell Carcinoma and Diagnostic Methods

The mean size of the tumors found was 4.0 ± 2.7 cm in diameter (Fig. 48). Small tumors of less than 2 cm are difficult to detect by either CT scan or ultrasonography (Fig. 49), but such tumors have been detected by the full use of imaging techniques. However, many renal cell carcinomas have only been detected after they have grown to a very large size.

5 Differences Between Japan and the United States

We compared renal cell carcinomas in dialysis patients in Japan and the United States. The incidence was 113 per 100 000 patient-years in the U.S. [91], but was slightly higher at 193 per 100 000 patient-years in Japan [63].The incidence of renal cell

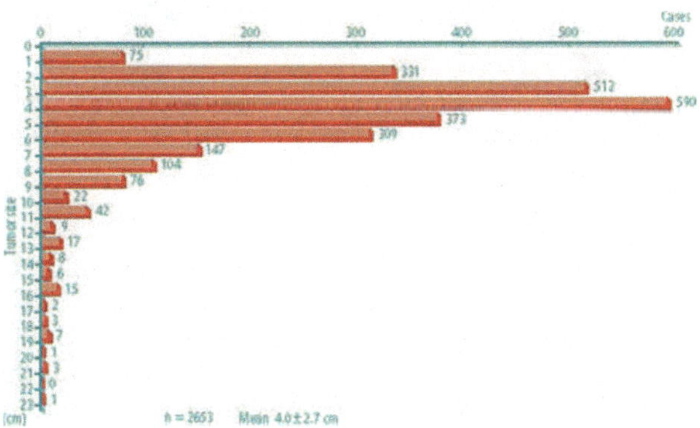

FIG. 48. Size of renal cell carcinoma

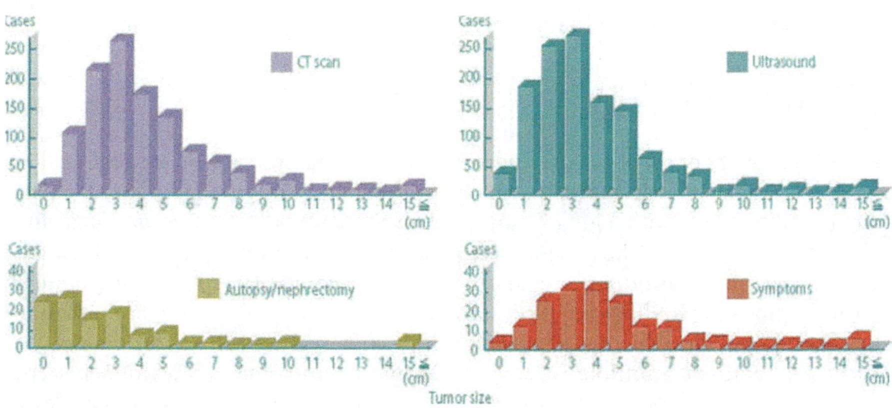

FIG. 49. Size of renal cell carcinoma and diagnostic aids

TABLE 12. Comparison of renal cell carcinoma in dialysis patients in Japan and in the United States

	General population	Dialysis patients	SIR (standardized incidence ratio)
Japan	$3/_{100\,000}$	$193/_{100\,000}$*	14.3–17.1*
USA	$7/_{100\,000}$	$113/_{100\,000}$**	3.7**

*, Questionnaire study in 2004
**, Maisonneuve P: Lancet 354:93, 1999

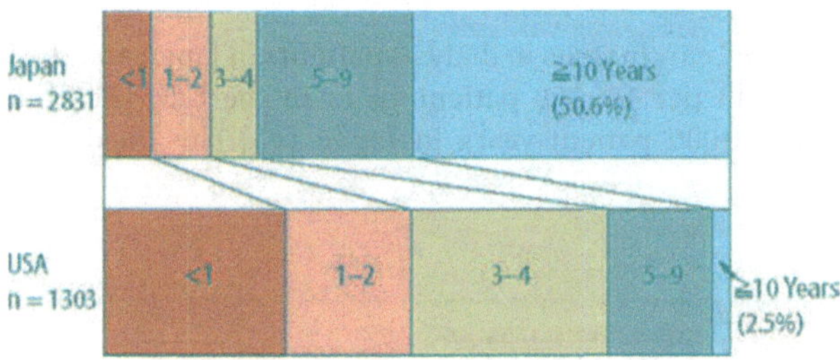

FIG. 50. Comparison of the duration of dialysis (years) in renal cell carcinoma patients between Japan and the United States

carcinomas in dialysis patients was 3.7 times higher than that in the general population in the U.S., and 14–17 times higher in Japan (Table 12). The prevalence (number of cancer patients/number of all patients) was 0.46%–0.49% in the U.S. [91], but was 0.85%–1.45% in Japan. The increase in renal cell carcinomas with the duration of dialysis from 5–10 years to 10 years or longer was greater in Japan than in the U.S. [84]. However, the most striking difference between the two countries was observed in the duration of dialysis in renal cell carcinoma patients. This was 10 years or longer in only 2.5% of patients in the U.S. [91] but in 50.6% of patients in Japan (Fig. 50). In addition, the age at which dialysis was initiated was 34 years or less in 5.2% of the renal cell carcinoma patients in the U.S., but in 28.2% of patients in Japan.

6 Characteristics

The characteristics of renal cell carcinoma in dialysis patients may be summarized as follows. (1) Renal cell carcinoma occurs more frequently in younger patients, male patients, and patients with a long history of dialysis. (2) It is often asymptomatic and difficult to diagnose. (3) The prognosis is relatively good, but metastasis is occasionally observed, and death due to renal cancer is not rare. (4) Histologically, granular cell carcinoma and papillary renal cell carcinoma are noted more frequently than in the general population due to their relationships with cysts. (5) Renal cell carcinoma is often bilateral and multiple [62,92]. According to outcome studies of renal cell carcinoma [11,58,93], renal cell carcinoma was bilateral in 78 (14.5%) of 539 cases. (6) Renal cell carcinoma occurs less frequently after renal transplantation because of the regression of cysts. However, the effects of immunosuppressants cannot be ignored. In Japan, renal cell carcinoma is the most frequent malignant tumor diagnosed after renal transplantation.

From these characteristics, (1) being a young male, (2) having received dialysis over a long period, and (3) enlargement of the kidneys due to acquired renal cysts are considered to be risk factors for renal cell carcinoma.

7 Diagnosis

Since renal cell carcinoma is rarely symptomatic, dialysis patients must be screened periodically by imaging techniques to ensure its early detection. Imaging studies are essential when gross hematuria is observed [11,93,94].

7.1 Ultrasonography

Ultrasonography is performed first for imaging screening because it is not invasive, can readily be repeated, and is inexpensive [95]. Its disadvantages are that the effectiveness is largely operator-dependent, that delineation of small tumors is difficult, that renal cell carcinomas are imaged as masses with an internal echo while cysts have no internal echo, and that small kidneys are difficult to image if there is much fat (Table 13). In Figs. 51 and 52, a tumor 4 cm in diameter is clearly delineated, and the renal cell carcinoma is imaged as a mass with an internal echo. However, the detection of renal cell carcinomas of 2 cm or less in diameter is occasionally difficult, and depends on the operator's skill. Because of these disadvantages of ultrasonography, a CT scan is more reliable for the diagnosis of renal cell carcinoma [11,93].

7.2 CT Scan

The point of diagnosis of renal cell carcinoma by CT scan is to examine whether there is a mass with the same X-ray absorption value as renal parenchyma [11,96] (Cases 7 and 16) (see Figs. 53,54,85,103). If part of the kidney has the same X-ray absorption value as the parenchyma in a patient with a long history of dialysis, and if it retains

TABLE 13. The use of ultrasonography for the diagnosis of renal cell carcinoma in dialysis patients

1. Renal cell carcinoma appears as a mass with an internal echo
2. A mass which appears "intermediate" by a CT scan is a hemorrhagic or high-protein-containing cyst if there is no echo in the mass by ultrasonography. Renal cell carcinoma and hemorrhagic cysts can be differentiated using ultrasonography
3. However, 50% of hemorrhagic cysts may show an internal echo if they contain blood clots. In this situation it is difficult to differentiate between renal cell carcinoma and hemorrhagic (blood clot) cysts
4. Detection of cysts by ultrasound is more reliable than by CT scan. The sensitivity of the detection of renal cell carcinoma in dialysis patients is lower by ultrasound scan than by CT scan
5. Detection of renal cell carcinoma by ultrasonography is operator-dependent. A comparison of images between the current year and the previous year is more difficult in ultrasonography than in CT scan
6. Contrast (Levovist)-enhanced ultrasonography is a promising development for the future

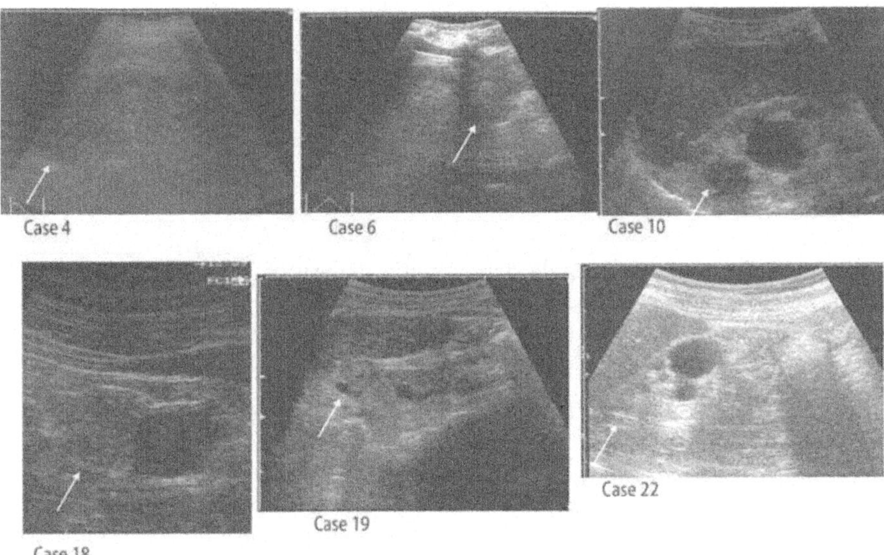

FIG. 51. Ultrasound findings of renal cell carcinoma (*arrows*), 1

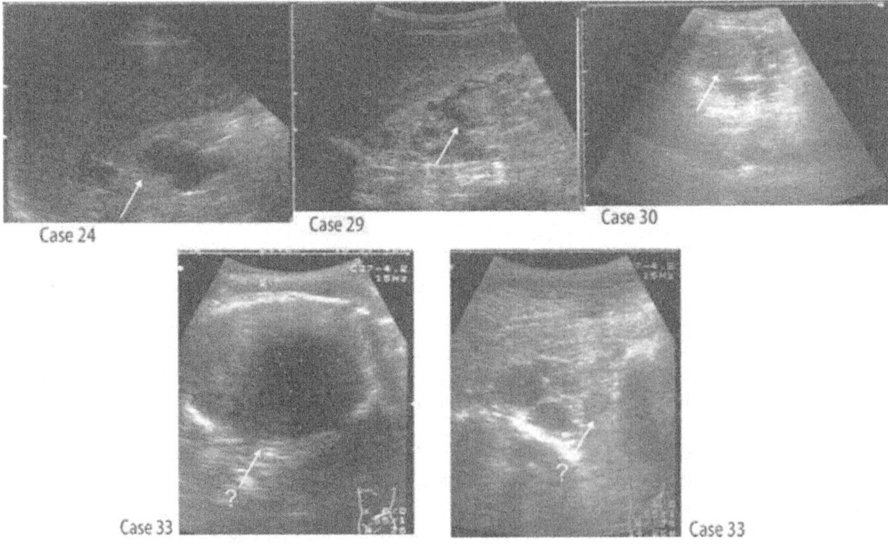

FIG. 52. Ultrasound findings of renal cell carcinoma (*arrows*), 2

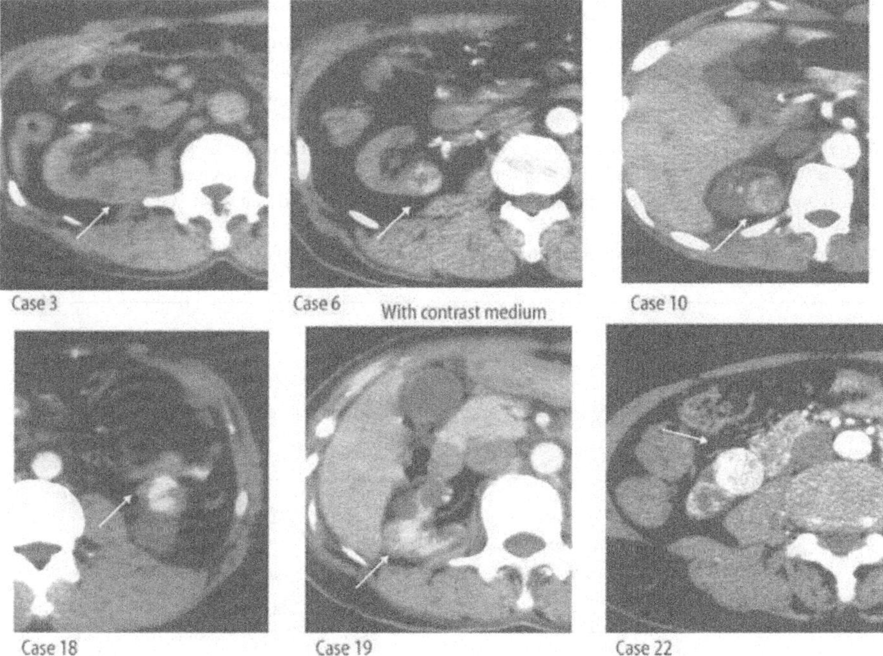

FIG. 53. CT images of renal cell carcinoma (*arrows*), 1. Renal cell carcinoma is often hypervascular in patients with a short history of dialysis (≤10 years). The tumor in Case 3 was not proved to be a hypervascular tumor because of the poor timing of the procedure (CT in Case 6: Reproduced from [6], by permission of Oxford University Press)

a normal thickness, the finding is clearly abnormal, and this is an important point for the detection of a small renal cell carcinoma (Table 14). In addition, if a suspicious mass is detected by plain CT, whether or not there is blood flow (contrast enhancement) in the mass must be examined by dynamic CT [97], because there is no blood flow in the mass and no contrast enhancement is observed if the mass is a hemorrhagic cyst or a cyst filled with a high-protein fluid.

In patients with a short history of dialysis, renal cell carcinoma is often imaged as a mass projecting from the renal margin (Figs. 53 and 55), and is relatively easy to diagnose. However, diagnosis is difficult in patients with a long history of dialysis because a renal cell carcinoma is often surrounded by many cysts, and located in the interior of the kidney without any irregularity of the renal margin or protrusion of the tumor on the renal surface [98] (Figs. 54, 55, 103). In male patients in particular cysts occur in large numbers, and renal cell carcinomas are buried in these cysts, so they are very difficult to diagnose even by CT scan, and often are only detected after they have grown to a large size. Dynamic helical CT rather than delayed CT should be used for a definitive preoperative diagnosis. Dynamic helical CT is particularly useful for the examination of early contrast enhancement [99]. Figure 56 shows a mass that clearly showed contrast enhancement on dynamic CT, and was diagnosed as a

TABLE 14. The use of CT scan for the diagnosis of renal cell carcinoma in dialysis patients

1. CT scan is more reliable than ultrasound for detecting renal cell carcinoma in dialysis patients
2. A mass with an isodensity which is the same as that of renal parenchyma should be suspected to be a renal cell carcinoma. If the contrast enhancement of a mass is more than 10–20 HU by an enhanced helical CT scan, then it is a renal cell carcinoma
3. A large renal cell carcinoma often shows calcifications in the center or in the peripheral area, and there is also an irregular margin and inhomogeneous enhancement in the tumor
4. The image of a CT scan is not operator-dependent, and therefore it can easily be compared with the previous CT scan
5. Renal cell carcinoma in dialysis patients is often multicentric and bilateral. A CT scan is the most suitable in this situation

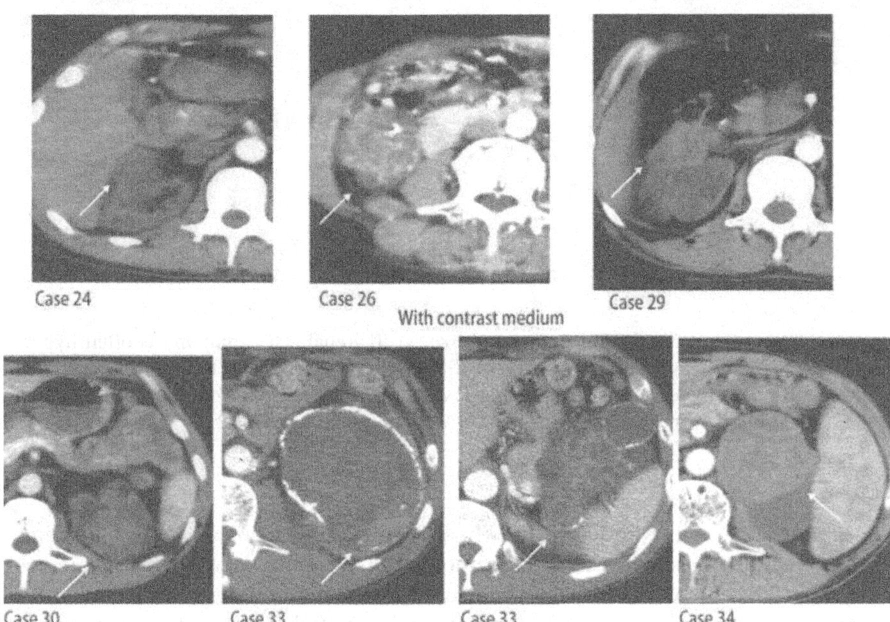

FIG. 54. CT images of renal cell carcinoma (*arrows*), 2. Renal cell carcinoma is often hypo-vascular in patients with a long history of dialysis (>10 years) (CT in Case 29: Reproduced from [6], by permission of Oxford University Press)

hypervascular renal cell carcinoma. The dynamic CT curve also showed contrast enhancement in the vascular phase in the area of the tumor.

Some renal cell carcinomas of dialysis patients show contrast enhancement but not a very high enhancement rate, i.e., hypovascular tumors in the angiographic term. As shown in Fig. 57, contrast enhancement is smaller in papillary renal cell carcinoma than in nonpapillary renal cell carcinoma. In such cases, the CT value of the mass must be determined by dynamic CT before the administration of the contrast medium and in the arterial phase, and blood flow is judged to be present in the mass if a contrast enhancement of 10–20 HU or greater is observed in the arterial phase (see

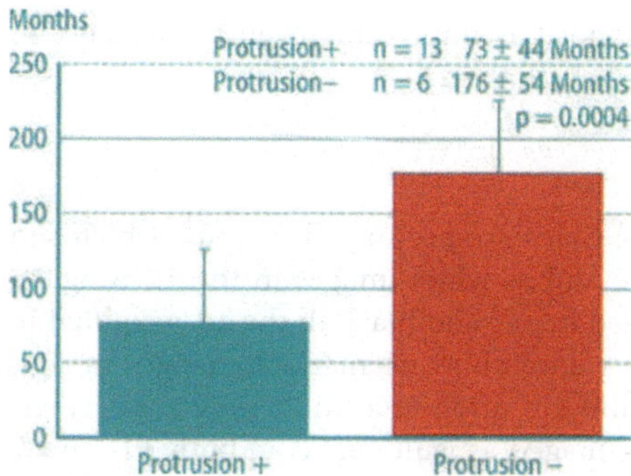

FIG. 55. Duration of dialysis and protrusion of renal cell carcinoma from the renal margin. Renal cell carcinoma often protrudes from the renal margin in patients with a short history of dialysis, but not often in those with a long history of dialysis

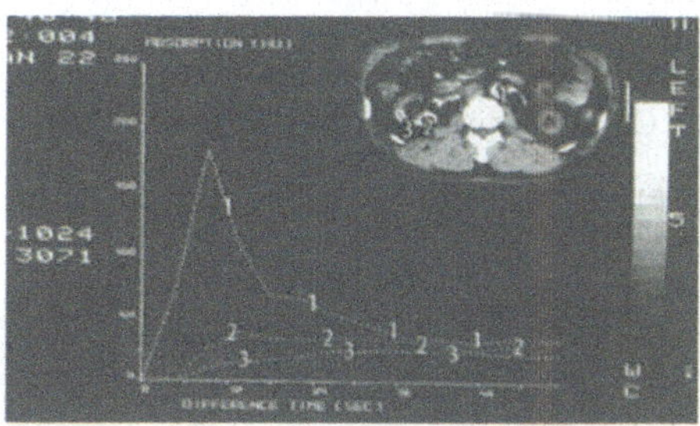

FIG. 56. Contrast enhancement of renal cell carcinoma on dynamic CT. Contrast enhancement is more intense in renal cell carcinoma (2) than in the renal parenchyma (3)

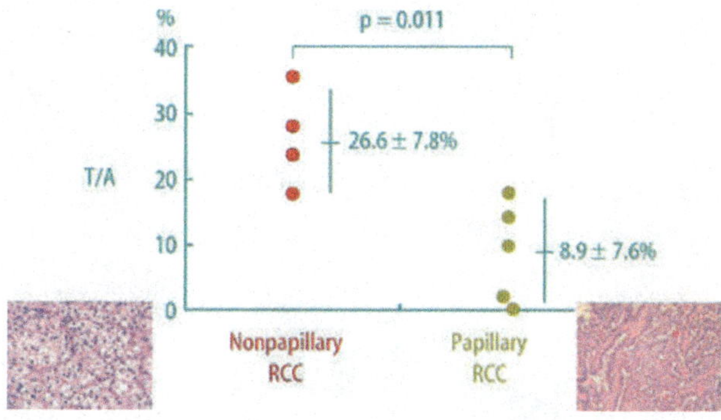

FIG. 57. Ratio of contrast enhancement of the tumor relative to that of the aorta (T/A). Comparison between nonpapillary renal cell carcinoma and papillary renal cell carcinoma

Fig. 53, 54). If the diagnosis is impossible even by helical CT, magnetic resonance imaging (MRI) must be performed.

7.3 MRI

By MRI, the T1 and T2 times are prolonged in cysts, which show as black images in the T1-weighted image and as white images in the T2-weighted image. Fat appears white in the T1-weighted image and black in the T2-weighted image. In addition, the renal parenchyma and tumor show no marked changes in signal intensity in T1- or T2-weighted images, and are often imaged as gray areas (Figs. 58–61). In addition, hemorrhagic cysts are imaged as white areas in both T1- and T2-weighted images if the hemorrhage is fresh, but are imaged as areas with intermediate signal intensity in the T1-weighted image and as black areas in the T2-weighted image if the hemorrhage is old. Therefore, hemorrhagic cysts can be excluded if gray lesions are observed in the T2-weighted image [98,100]. However, a diagnosis of renal cell carcinoma is often difficult by MRI alone, because there are few findings which are specific to renal cell carcinoma. In such cases, the accuracy of the diagnosis is further improved by the concomitant use of dynamic MRI with gadolinium diethylenetriaminopentoacetic acid (Gd-DTPA).

Some examples of MR images are now presented. In Case 24 (see Fig. 119), since the findings on dynamic CT or ultrasonography were not sufficiently convincing, we

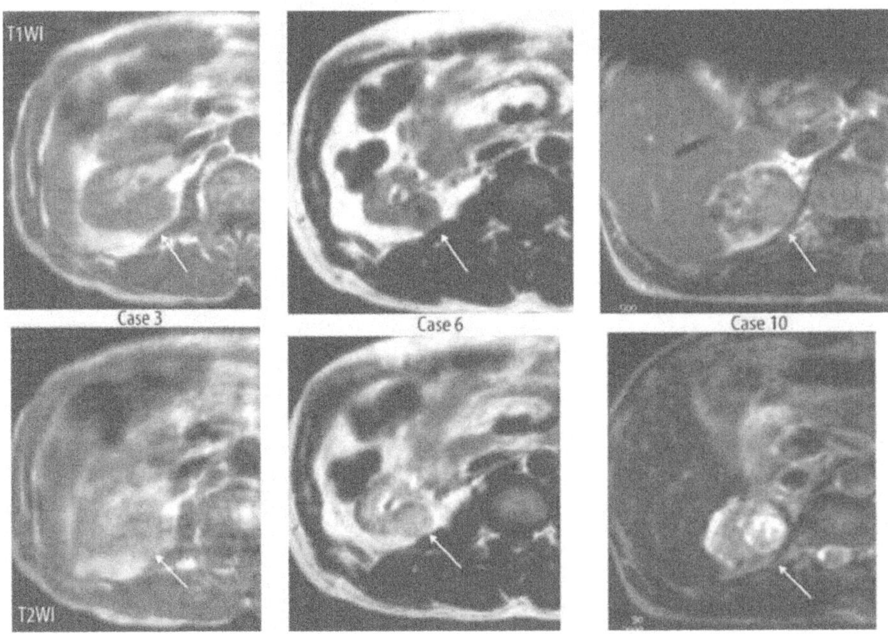

Fig. 58. Magnetic resonance (MR) images of renal cell carcinoma (*arrows*), 1. The signal intensity of the renal tumor is close to that of the renal parenchyma

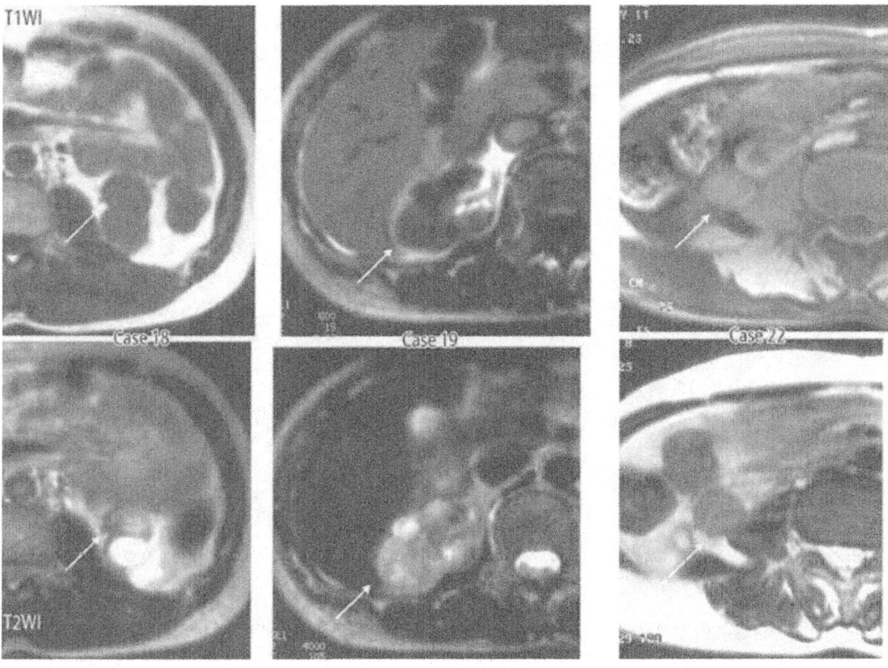

Fig. 59. MR images of renal cell carcinoma (*arrows*), 2. Renal cell carcinoma is delineated as a gray area, particularly in T2WI, unlike cysts, which appear as white areas. This difference is important when renal cell carcinoma is surrounded by cysts

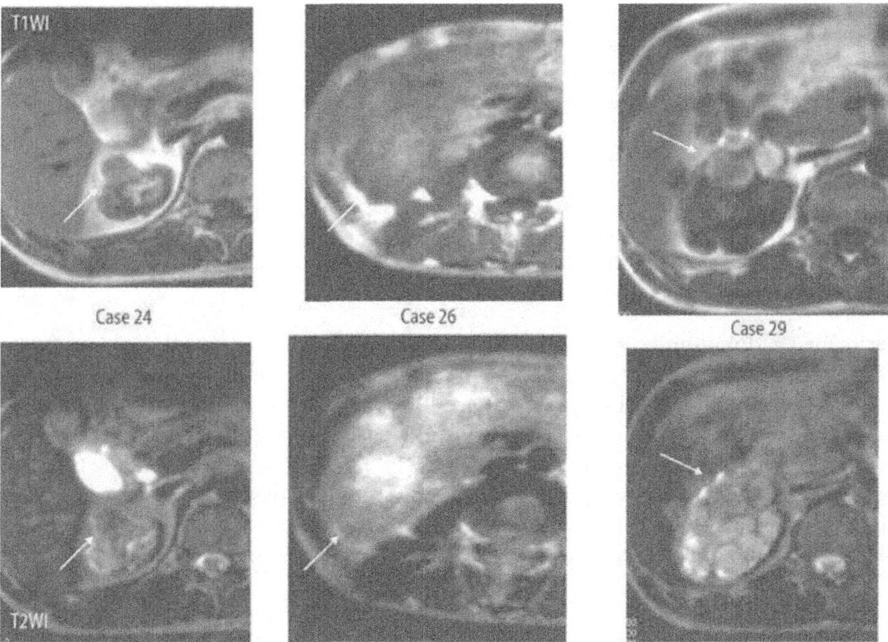

Fig. 60. MR images of renal cell carcinoma (*arrows*), 3. The gray lesion in the *right* T2WI (Case 29) is particularly important

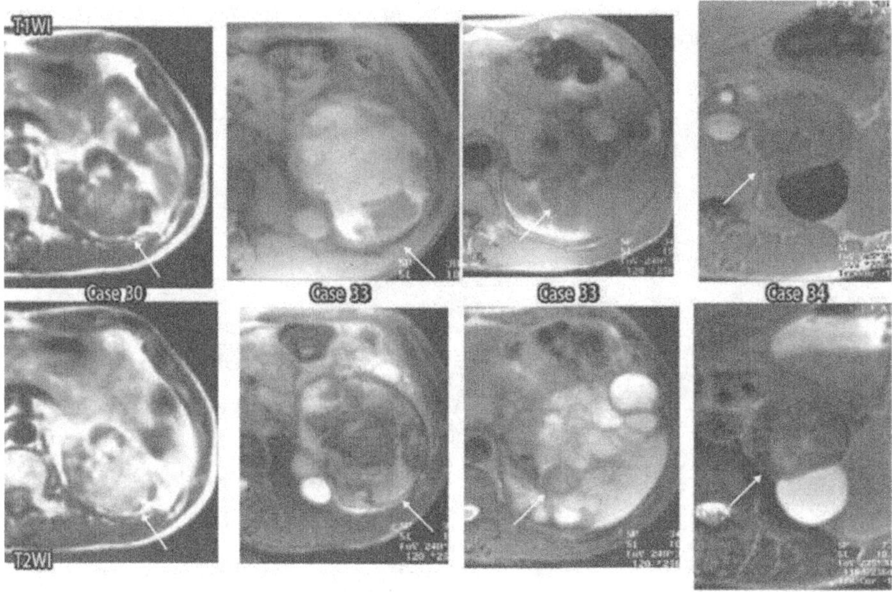

FIG. 61. MR images of renal cell carcinoma (*arrows*), 4. In patients with a long history of dialysis, cysts often occur in large numbers, renal cell carcinoma may be surrounded by cysts, and renal cell carcinoma may develop in the calcified walls of hematomas. Note the gray lesion in the second T2WI from the right (Case 33)

TABLE 15. Summary of the use of MRI for the diagnosis of renal cell carcinoma in dialysis patients

1. MRI is used when a diagnosis of renal cell carcinoma is equivocal by enhanced helical CT scan
2. A renal cell carcinoma surrounded by extensive cystic changes may be diagnosed by MRI
3. Renal cell carcinoma is strongly suspected when there is a region of intermediate intensity by T2 weighted images (T2WI)
4. The age of fresh or old bleeding may be diagnosed by MRI
5. If a mass shows enhancement by gadolinium–diethylenetriaminopentoacetic acid (Gd–DTPA)-enhanced MRI, a diagnosis of renal cell carcinoma can be made. However, it should be noted that some tumors reveal only a little enhancement

performed gadolinium DTPA-enhanced MRI. This showed an area with clear contrast enhancement, and we could operate on this patient with confidence.

The upper photographs in Figs. 58–61 are T1-weighted images of 12 of my renal cell carcinoma patients. The lower photographs in Figs. 58–61 are T2-weighted images of the same patients. The signal intensity was high in parts of the tumors, but the tumors were mostly difficult to distinguish from the surrounding tissues. In some cases, the diagnosis appears to be easier by T2-weighted images (Figs. 60 and 61) when a renal cell carcinoma is surrounded by cysts. Table 15 summarizes the MRI findings.

7.4 Difficulties in the Diagnosis of Renal Cell Carcinoma in Dialysis Patients [98]

1. Renal cell carcinoma is often asymptomatic and can be overlooked without screening.

2. Renal cell carcinoma can be diagnosed relatively easily in patients with a short duration of dialysis, because it is observed as a protrusion from the renal margin. However, in patients with a long duration of dialysis, it is concealed by many cysts and is difficult to diagnose. T2-weighted MRI may be useful for the diagnosis of renal cell carcinoma surrounded by cysts. However, the diagnosis becomes easier 1 month or longer after renal transplantation because of regression of the cysts.

3. Since papillary renal cell carcinoma is often a hypovascular tumor, it is difficult to diagnose. Papillary renal cell carcinoma located in the hematoma wall is even more difficult to diagnose. Its differentiation from a hemorrhagic cyst is important.

4. Contrast-enhanced helical CT is the best for the diagnosis of renal cell carcinoma. However, caution is necessary, because no contrast enhancement is observed in spindle cell carcinoma (sarcomatoid renal cell carcinoma), as mentioned below.

7.5 Screening

A flowchart for the detection of renal cell carcinoma is shown in Fig. 62. In addition to screening symptomatic patients, we consider that periodic screening is necessary once a year for asymptomatic male patients, and once every 2 years for asymptomatic

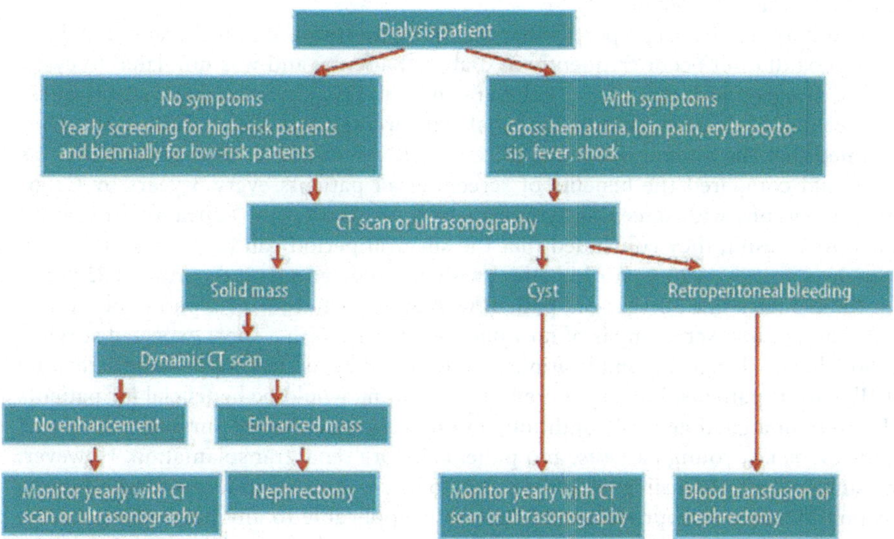

FIG. 62. Methods for screening diseased kidneys for renal cell carcinoma, examinations, and treatments (Reproduced from [11], with permission from S. Karger AG)

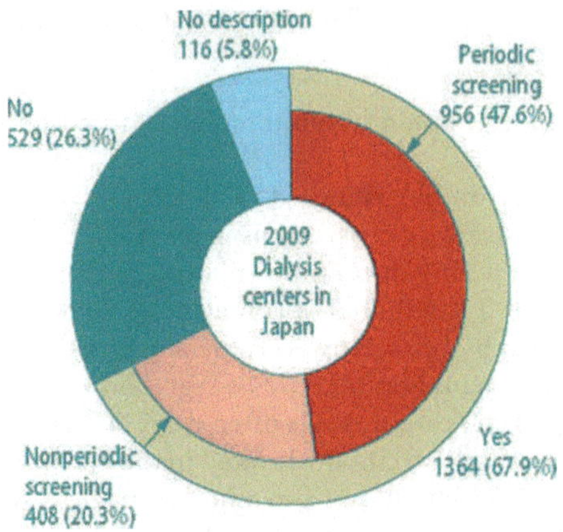

FIG. 63. Screening dialysis patients for renal cell carcinoma

female patients and patients who have undergone renal transplantation [11]. Questions concerning screening for renal cell carcinoma were incorporated in a questionnaire survey of dialysis centers in Japan. It was found that some screening was performed at 1 364 dialysis facilities (67.9%), and periodic screening was performed at 956 facilities (47.6%) [84] (Fig. 63). The frequency of screening was once a year in 78.9% of the facilities and twice a year or more in 18.3%. Screening was performed by ultrasonography at 42% of the facilities, by CT scan at 23%, and by both ultrasonography and CT scan at 21%.

Chandhoke et al. [101] reported that screening was unnecessary, because renal cell carcinoma did not occur frequently in dialysis patients, and was unrelated to cysts, but we disagree with this view [102]. Sarasin et al. [103] evaluated the effectiveness of screening of dialysis patients for renal cell carcinoma by decision analysis. They assumed that the annual incidence of renal cell carcinoma in dialysis patients was 0.9%, and compared the benefits of screening all patients every 3 years by CT or ultrasonography with screening symptomatic patients after the appearance of symptoms. As a result, they concluded that the survival period can be prolonged for 1.6 years by screening a 20-year-old patient with an expected survival period of 25 years, but for 4–5 days in a 58-year-old patient with an expected survival period of 5 years, and reported that screening is of no value for patients with a short expected survival period due to old age or complications. Therefore, they did not support the screening of all dialysis patients, but considered that screening would be beneficial for patients who were in a good general condition, and had a long expected survival period and many cysts, i.e., young patients, and patients before renal transplantation. However, the simulation by Sarasin et al. [103] needs to be reevaluated in terms of whether the assumption used is appropriate, whether it is applicable to any particular country, and when the expected survival period for dialysis patients can be extended in the future.

Furthermore, Denton et al. [56] indicated that prospective studies are necessary in order to evaluate the usefulness of screening high-risk patients. Choyke [104] reported

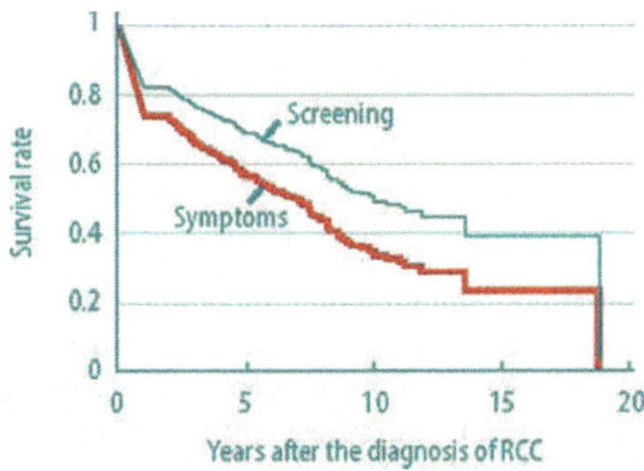

FIG. 64. Comparison of the survival rate between patients in whom renal cell carcinoma was detected because of their symptoms and those in whom it was detected by screening (deaths from all causes) (p = 0.0119) (Reproduced from [105], with permission from Blackwell Publishing)

that the screening of most patients is recommended in countries where the expected survival period of dialysis patients is long, such as Japan.

According to our evaluation, the outcomes of treatment were better in patients whose diagnosis of renal cell carcinoma was by screening than in those who were diagnosed by examinations after the appearance of symptoms [105] (Fig. 64).

Also on the basis of the results for Japanese dialysis patients obtained by our questionnaire survey in 2002, Brown observed in the editorial of the May 2004 issue of *Nephron*: "There is no doubt that such screening should take place. Common sense should be used to select patients for screening and to thereby avoid unnecessary stress and anxiety in patients at low risk or those who are unlikely to benefit as their survival is not going to be extended by the finding and removal of a renal tumor" [106]. Apart from the frequency, we agree that this principle of screening is appropriate at present [90].

8 Treatment

Nephrectomy after early diagnosis is considered to be the only treatment for renal cell carcinoma [11,14]. Only the kidney with the tumor should be resected, and the other kidney should be examined by imaging techniques once every 3–6 months. The surgery may be simple nephrectomy or radial nephrectomy, but the less invasive peritoneoscopic nephrectomy, laparoscopic nephrectomy, and retroperitoneoscopic nephrectomy have been performed recently [107–109]. According to one questionnaire survey [58], simple nephrectomy was performed in 283 patients (54.4%), and radical nephrectomy in 237 patients (45.6%); nephrectomy was unilateral in 377 patients (78.9%) and bilateral in 101 patients (21.1%).

Interferon is used occasionally as an adjuvant therapy. Out of 491 patients, 410 were observed, 68 (13.8%) were administered interferon, and 13 received other treatments [58].

Regarding surgical indications, nephrectomy should be performed if a vascularized tumor of any size with an X-ray value similar to that of the renal parenchyma is detected by dynamic CT, on condition that the patient tolerates the surgery. At present, usually only the kidney with the tumor is resected.

9 Prognosis

The prognosis of renal cell carcinoma is generally good, but occasional poor outcomes are possible. According to the results of a questionnaire survey, metastasis was observed in 15% of the patients (during a follow-up for a mean of 1 year), and the sites of metastasis included bone, liver, lung, lymph nodes, and brain. Renal cell carcinomas with metastases are larger than those without metastases, but even renal cell carcinomas 1.2 cm and 1.5 cm in diameter were reported to have metastasized [4]. According to the first report on prognosis by Matson and Cohen [110], the 5-year survival rate of dialysis patients with renal cell carcinoma was 35%, which was the same as that of nondialysis patients with renal cell carcinoma.

We studied the outcomes of 848 patients in 9 questionnaire surveys [58]. In these patients, the mean duration of dialysis was 10 years, the mean age at the diagnosis of renal cell carcinoma was 53 years, and the mean follow-up period after the diagnosis was 4.7 years. The observed 5-year survival rate was 64.0% (10-year survival rate 47.2%, 15-year survival rate 35.0%). The 5-year survival rate of patients who did not develop renal cell carcinoma was 78.1% [58] (Fig. 65). On closer analysis, the survival rate of patients with renal cell carcinoma was found to have decreased markedly within 2 years after the diagnosis, and remained 14% lower than the survival rate of patients without renal cell carcinoma 2–6 years after the diagnosis. These parallel changes in the survival rate in the two groups indicate that, if treatment (surgery) is performed appropriately, renal cell carcinoma is unlikely to affect the outcome

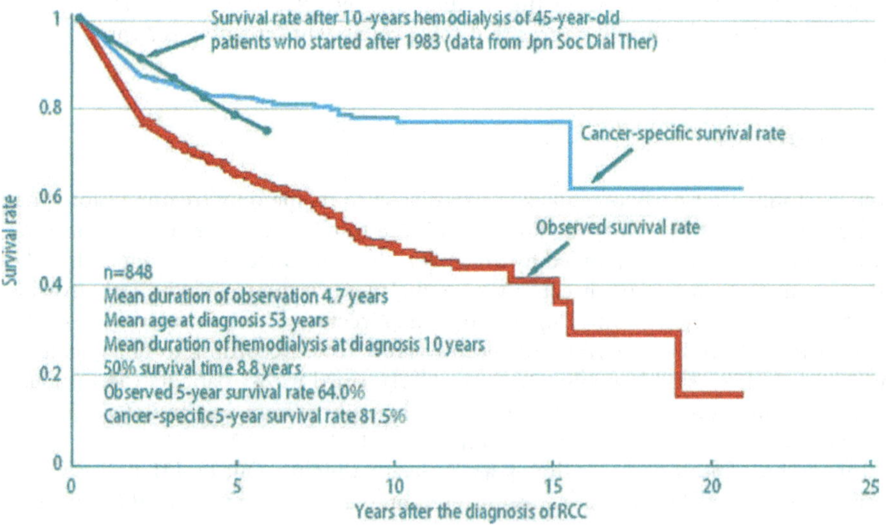

FIG. 65. Observed survival rate and cancer-specific survival rate in dialysis patients with renal cell carcinoma (Reproduced from [58], with permission)

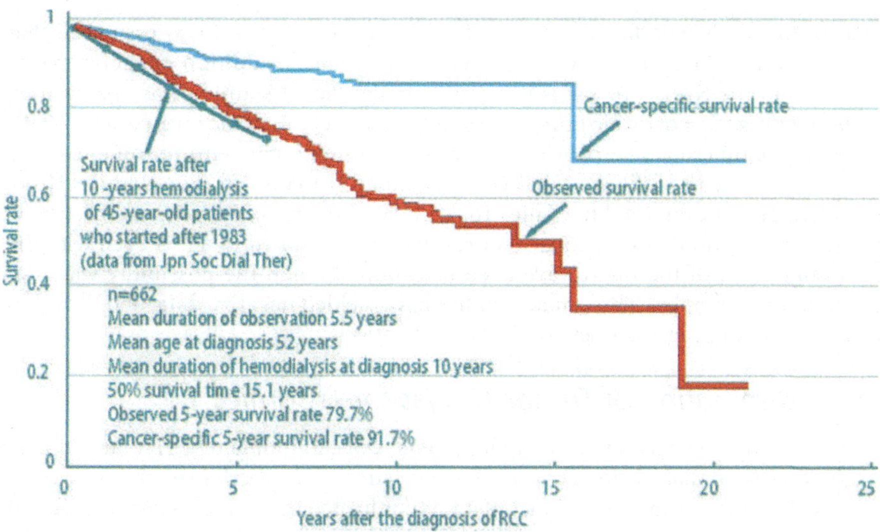

FIG. 66. Observed survival rate and cancer-specific survival rate in dialysis patients with renal cell carcinoma (surgical cases) (Reproduced from [58], with permission)

thereafter. Regarding the renal cell carcinoma-specific survival rates, the 5-year, 10-year, and 15-year survival rates were 81.5%, 76.5%, and 76.0%, respectively.

Of the 761 patients who mentioned their history of surgery in the questionnaire, 662 (87%) had undergone surgery. In these patients, the mean age at the diagnosis of renal cell carcinoma was 52 years, the mean duration of dialysis was 10 years, and the mean postoperative follow-up period was 5.5 years. The observed 5-year survival rate was 79.7%, which was close to the 78.1% of those who did not develop renal cell carcinoma (Fig. 66). The cancer-specific 5-year survival rate was 91.7%. These results suggest that the outcome is dependent on the age and stage of the tumor at diagnosis, and that it is poorer as these are more advanced [58].

From our experience, we consider that the mortality rate due to renal cell carcinoma, i.e., its prognosis, is similar in dialysis patients and in the general population if the comparison is made between grade- and stage-matched subjects. However, many investigators consider that the prognosis of renal cell carcinoma is better in dialysis patients than in the general population [11,111,112]. It is likely that this is primarily because renal cell carcinoma tends to be detected in an earlier stage in dialysis patients due to screening [105].

10 Etiology

10.1 History of Research into the Etiology

I first evaluated whether there were mutagenic factors in cyst fluid in 1980. I requested the National Cancer Center to examine this by the Ames test, but cyst fluid was negative for mutagenic factors. An examination at our university also showed that the EGF level in the cyst fluid was not abnormally high. In addition, no abnormality was noted in the N-, H-, or K-ras gene, and no significant staining was observed by in situ hybridization of cystic fibrosis transmembrane conductance regulator (CFTR). Moreover, no tuberous sclerosis complex 2 (TCS2) mutation of chromosome 16 could be demonstrated in papillary renal cell carcinoma (in collaboration with A. Hino, 1996). I therefore examined trisomies 16, 7, and 17 in renal cell carcinoma tissues by in situ hybridization, but no consistent results were obtained by FISH even with the concomitant use of the microwave oven method, although the possibility was suggested in some samples. Thus, many studies have yielded negative data, and there has been no marked progress in etiological investigations.

10.2 Examination of Tumor Tissues for Trisomies

Figure 67 shows the karyotype of papillary renal cell carcinoma in a 41-year-old man who had received dialysis for 11 years. The presence of renal cell carcinoma was suspected before renal transplantation, but it was confirmed by the regression of acquired renal cysts after transplantation (Case 24), and right nephrectomy was performed 5 months after transplantation. Histologically, the tumor was a papillary renal cell carcinoma, and its karyotype was 48, X, −Y, +5, +16, +20 instead of trisomy 7 (+7) or trisomy 17 (+17).

Figure 68 summarizes the karyotypes of papillary renal cell carcinomas in our 15 cases and 10 cases in the literature [6]. Trisomy 16 (+16), trisomy 7 (+7), and Y deletion were observed frequently, but trisomy 17 (+17) was not frequent, and the karyotypes of papillary renal cell carcinomas in dialysis patients appeared to be slightly different from those in the general population [113–120].

Next, we examined 3p deletion in 4 of our patients with nonpapillary renal cell carcinomas. The 3p deletion, i.e., the deletion of a tumor suppressor gene, was observed in 3 of the 4 patients, and loss of heterozygosity (LOH) was noted in 3p21.3, 3p14.2, 5q21, and 17p13, 17p13.3. However, their karyotypes did not appear to differ from those of nonpapillary renal cell carcinomas in the general population [117] (Fig. 69).

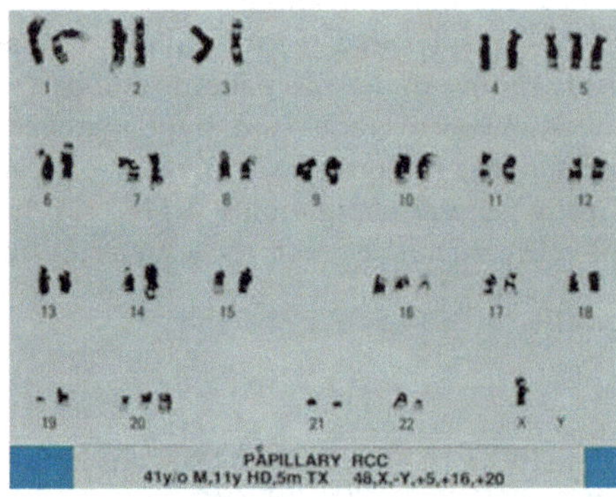

FIG. 67. Karyotype of papillary renal cell carcinoma. The karyotype of this case was 48,X, −Y,+5,+16,+20, and no +7 and +17 were observed (Reproduced from [118], with permission from Elsevier Inc.)

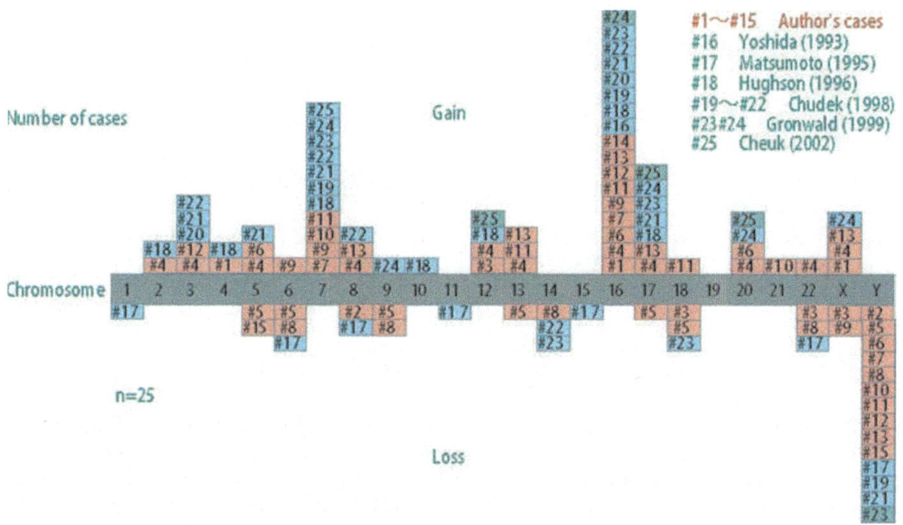

FIG. 68. Changes in the number of chromosomes in papillary renal cell carcinoma (Reproduced from [6], with permission by permission of Oxford University Press)

	Case1	Case2	Case3	Case4
Age/sex	71-year-old male	69-year-old male	39-year-old male	43-year-old male
Duration of dialysis	2 months	1 year 2 months	6 months dialysis, 8 years 4 months after transplantation	2 years 2 months
Metastasis		Metastasis		
3p21.3	LOH	LOH		
3p14.2			LOH	
5q21	LOH			LOH
17p13		LOH		
17p13.3		LOH		

FIG. 69. Search for loss of heterozygosity (LOH) by restriction fragment length polymorphism (RFLP) in dialysis patients who developed nonpapillary renal cell carcinoma (Reproduced from [117], with permission)

Subsequently, we studied the LOH of von Hippel–Lindau (VHL) disease gene at 3p25, which we had not done previously. In a joint study with Yoshida et al. [121] of VHL mutations for clear cell carcinoma, we detected the LOH of VHL (3p25) in 3 of 8 patients with clear cell carcinoma. By microsatellite allelotyping using D3S1038, tumors that showed the 618delA mutation (Fig. 70) were detected. However, no c-Met mutation was noted in the 6 patients with papillary renal cell carcinoma.

Thus, the karyotypes of renal cell carcinomas of dialysis patients appear to be mainly similar to those of the general population, and this is also true from a molecular biological viewpoint, but there do seem to be a few differences, and further research is necessary.

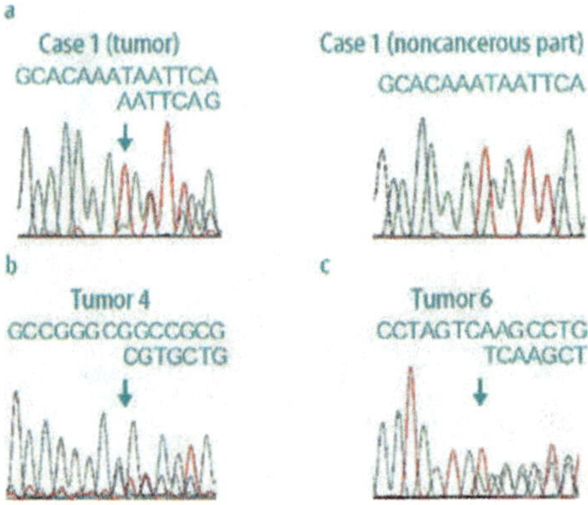

FIG. 70. von Hippel-Lindau disease (VHL) gene mutations in nonpapillary renal cell carcinoma (clear cell carcinoma). **a** The tumor in Case 1 showed 618delA mutation, but the noncancerous parts showed the normal sequence. **b** Tumor 4 showed 386del 10bp mutation. **c** Tumor 6 showed 723–724insTC mutation (Reproduced from [121], with permission from John Wiley & Sons, Inc.)

Recently, Cheuk et al. [113] studied the karyotypes of areas other than renal cell carcinoma in one patient. As a result, the karyotype was +7 in the papillary tuft, +7,+17 in the cribriform part, +7,+12,+17,+20,+Y in atypical cysts, and +7,+12,+17,+20 in renal cell carcinoma. These findings are of profound interest if chromosomes 7 and 17 are related to growth factors such as EGFR and c-erbB2 [60].

We now look at research from some other facilities into the proliferation of cyst epithelial cells. Mutation of the p32 gene was rarely observed in renal cell carcinomas of dialysis patients [122]. In an early stage of renal cell carcinoma in dialysis patients, Connexin 32 (hypermethylation of its CpG island) may be acting as a tumor suppressor gene [123]. In the epithelium of atypical cysts, the HGF and c-met of its receptors were intensely stained, and the staining of Bcl-2 was similar [124].

Cytokines are related to the growth, differentiation, and apoptosis of cells, and the concentrations of IL-6, IL-8, and vascular endothelial growth factor (VEGF) were high in the cyst fluid of acquired cystic disease of the kidney [125]. Activator protein-1 (Jun, Fos) plays a central role in cytokine signal transmission, but phosphorylated c-Jun was positive in the epithelium of atypical cysts. Activation of c-Jun was also observed in early renal cell carcinomas. Therefore, stimulation by cytokines, including c-Jun, may be related to the proliferation of cyst epithelium [126].

Furthermore, Ca oxalate crystals are often found in tissues of acquired cystic disease of the kidney, and the plasma oxalate level is increased in dialysis patients. The differentiation and proliferation of proximal tubular cells associated with this increase in the oxalate level are related to oxalate deposition in the tumor [127]. Since renal cell carcinomas of dialysis patients often show Ca oxalate deposition, they are often bilateral or multicentric [128].

10.3 Hypotheses of the Pathogenic Mechanisms of Renal Cysts and Renal Cell Carcinoma

I have developed the following hypotheses concerning the pathogenic mechanisms of renal cysts and renal cell carcinoma (Fig. 71). In acquired cystic disease of the kidney, uremic metabolites increase with decreases in nephrons, and they affect the renal tubules. As a result, tubular cells change to poorly differentiated cells, causing abnormalities of proliferation, fluid secretion, and extracellular matrix, leading to cyst formation. As the production of uremic metabolites continues, they further act on the renal tubules along with growth factors and oxidative stress (free radicals). In addition, with decreases in active oxygen scavengers, a decrease in apoptosis, and impairment of the DNA repair mechanism, cysts develop into adenoma and renal cell carcinoma. A multistep pathogenic mechanism of renal cell carcinoma in dialysis patients that advances from cystic changes in tubular cells to atypical cysts, adenoma, and renal cell carcinoma has also been hypothesized by other investigators [3,129,130], but has not been validated (Fig. 71).

As for chromosomes, in the terminal stage of renal disease, changes occur in cell division, and acquired renal cysts develop. Numerical abnormalities in chromosomes may occur in cell division. In particular, I consider that trisomies 7 and 17 and Y chromosome deletion cause papillary adenoma, and trisomies 16, 12, and 20, in addition to these changes, cause papillary renal cell carcinoma. Uremic metabolites, local growth factors (overexpression of PDGF, EGF), mutagens in end-stage renal failure, and the impairment of the immunosurveillance mechanisms are also considered to change in this process, but this remains speculative. On the other hand, nonpapillary renal cell carcinoma is considered to occur, as in the general population, if structural

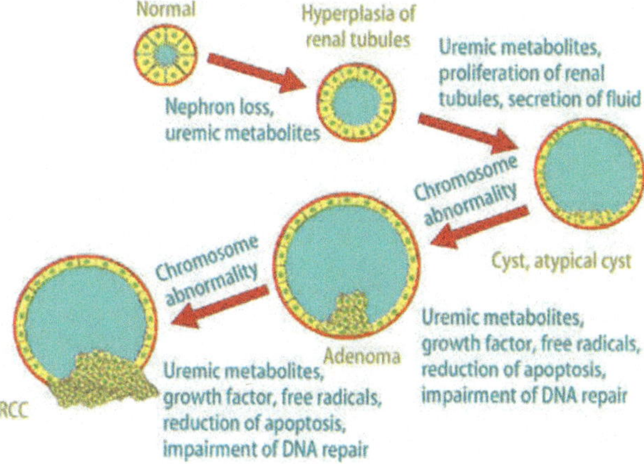

FIG. 71. Mechanism of the occurrence of acquired cystic disease of the kidney and renal cell carcinoma (hypothesis)

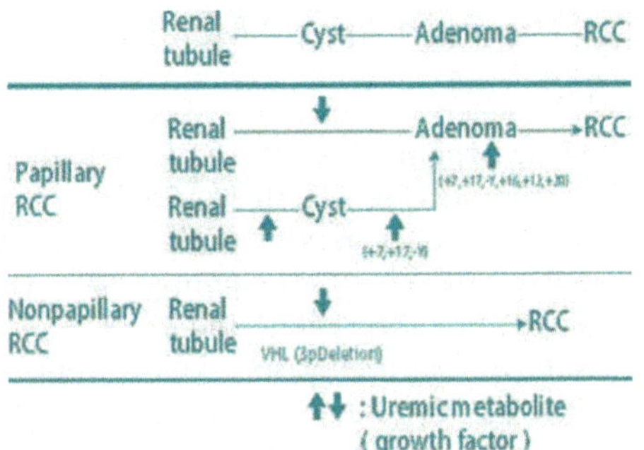

FIG. 72. Causes of renal cell carcinoma in dialysis patients seen from the viewpoint of chromosomal change

changes in chromosomes occur, particularly 3p deletion, i.e., deletion of a tumor suppressor gene (Fig. 72).

Gardner [131] suggested that the diseased kidneys of dialysis patients are "poststygian" kidneys, which alone are 100–150 years old irrespective of patient age. In such "poststygian" kidneys, vascular sclerosis, tubular proliferation, and the formation of cysts, adenoma, and cancer are observed. We speculate that cystic changes and malignant transformation occur in diseased kidneys with increases in the number of mitoses of tubular cells, which increase the possibility of DNA mutation and cause disorders of the immunosurveillance system.

Chapter 4
Atlas of Renal Cell Carcinoma in Our Dialysis Patients

Table 16 summarizes the renal cell carcinoma observed in our dialysis patients (Cases 1–34). The patients were listed in order of the duration of dialysis, and the images and pathological findings are presented in Figs. 73–140.

Case 1. A 63-year-old man with chronic glomerulonephritis 2 months before the initiation of dialysis and with a high creatinine level of 6.0 mg/dl. Clear cell carcinoma was detected before the initiation of dialysis by screening (Figs. 73 and 74). A mass protruding from the renal margin was detected by computed tomography (CT), and was diagnosed as renal cell carcinoma by magnetic resonance imaging (MRI). Nephrectomy was performed.

Case 2. A 72-year-old man with chronic glomerulonephritis and with a history of dialysis of 3 days. On dynamic helical CT, contrast enhancement was observed, and blood flow was shown in the tumor by Doppler ultrasonography. Nephrectomy was performed 3 days after the initiation of hemodialysis (clear cell carcinoma) (Figs. 75 and 76). A hypervascular tumor was found protruding from the renal margin.

Case 3. A 71-year-old man with possible chronic glomerulonephritis and with a history of dialysis of 2 months. A clear cell carcinoma was observed in this elderly patient with a short history of dialysis (Figs. 77 and 78). Although contrast enhancement was observed on dynamic CT, the timing for the demonstration of hypervascularity was missed.

Case 4. A 69-year-old man with possible chronic glomerulonephritis and with a history of dialysis of 1 year and 2 months. A clear cell carcinoma with metastasis was observed in this elderly patient with a short history of dialysis (Figs. 79 and 80). The tumor that protruded from the renal margin invaded surrounding tissues and metastasized to the lung.

Case 5. A 57-year-old man with chronic glomerulonephritis and with a history of dialysis of 1 year and 4 months. This was the smallest clear cell carcinoma and was 5 mm in diameter (Figs. 81 and 82). The small renal cell carcinoma that had developed in the cyst wall was diagnosed by dynamic CT.

Case 6. A 43-year-old man with chronic glomerulonephritis and with a history of dialysis of 2 years and 2 months. A clear cell carcinoma, 2 cm in diameter, was detected by CT screening (Figs. 83 and 84). The tumor protruded from the renal margin and was hypervascular.

TABLE 16. Our cases of renal cell carcinoma complicating end-stage renal disease (in order of the duration of dialysis)

	Age (years)	Sex	Primary disease	Gross hematuria	Diagnostic aids	Duration of dialysis
1	63	M	Chronic glomerulonephritis	–	CT screening	Minus 2 months
2	72	M	Chronic glomerulonephritis	–	CT screening	3 days
3	71	M	Suspected chronic glomerulonephritis	–	CT screening	2 months
4	69	M	Suspected chronic glomerulonephritis	–	CT screening	1 year 2 months
5	57	M	Chronic glomerulonephritis	+ (after diagnosis)	CT screening	1 year 4 months
6	43	M	Chronic glomerulonephritis	–	CT screening	2 years 2 months
7	63	F	Diabetic nephropathy	–	US screening	2 years 7 months
8	64	F	Diabetic nephropathy	–	CT screening	2 years 11 months
9	65	M	Diabetic nephropathy	–	Autopsy	4 years (CAPD)
10	44	M	Chronic glomerulonephritis	+	CT screening	5 years 5 months
11	28	M	Chronic glomerulonephritis (biopsy-proven)	–	CT screening	5 years 8 months
12	73	M	Chronic glomerulonephritis	–	CT screening	6 years
13	34	M	Chronic glomerulonephritis	–	CT screening	6 years 9 months (transplantation)
14	30	F	Chronic glomerulonephritis	–	CT screening	7 months 5 years 8 months (transplantation)
15	24	M	Rapidly progressive glomerulonephritis (biopsy-proven)	–	Symptom (fever)	6 years 11 months
16	31	M	Chronic glomerulonephritis	–	CT screening	7 years 8 months
17	28	F	Chronic glomerulonephritis	–	CT screening	8 years
18	39	M	Chronic glomerulonephritis (biopsy-proven)	–	CT screening	8 months 8 years 4 months (transplantation)
19	38	F	Toxemia of pregnancy	–	CT screening	8 years 11 months
20	62	M	Diabetic nephropathy	+ (after diagnosis)	CT screening	9 years 6 months (CAPD)
21	47	M	Chronic glomerulonephritis	–	Autopsy	10 years 6 months
22	55	F	Chronic glomerulonephritis	–	CT screening	11 years 3 months
23	41	M	Chronic glomerulonephritis	–	At nephrectomy (retroperitoneal bleeding)	11 years 3 months
24	41	M	Chronic glomerulonephritis (biopsy-proven)	–	CT screening	11 years 5 months (transplantation)
25	64	F	ADPKD	–	Autopsy	12 years 2 months
26	64	M	Suspected chronic glomerulonephritis	–	CT screening	13 years
27	68	M	Chronic glomerulonephritis	–	Autopsy	13 years 6 months
28	52	M	Chronic glomerulonephritis	–	CT screening	14 years 6 months
29	40	M	Chronic glomerulonephritis	–	CT screening	15 years 8 months
30	31	M	Chronic glomerulonephritis	–	CT screening	15 years 9 months
31	77	M	Chronic glomerulonephritis	–	Autopsy	11 years (CAPD) 8 years 10 months (HD)
32	59	M	Chronic glomerulonephritis	–	Symptom (anemia)	21 years 3 months
33	50	M	Chronic glomerulonephritis	+	Symptom	21 years 5 months
34	41	M	Chronic glomerulonephritis	–	CT screening	25 years 1 month

*Multifocal RCCs. RCC, renal cell carcinoma; CAPD, continuous ambulatory peritoneal dialysis

Tumor size (cm)	Pathology	Metastasis	Outcome (on January 15, 2006)
4.8	Clear cell carcinoma	−	Alive (1 year)
4.0	Clear cell carcinoma	−	Alive (0.8 year)
2.9	Clear cell carcinoma	−	Congestive heart failure (5.1 years)
6.0	Clear cell carcinoma	+ (lung)	Died of RCC (1.2 years)
0.5	Clear cell carcinoma	−	Alive (3.5 years)
2.0	Clear cell carcinoma	−	Alive (15.9 years)
3.8	Clear cell carcinoma	−	Alive (4.0 years)
3.0	Clear cell carcinoma	−	Alive (1.5 years)
1.0	Granular cell carcinoma	−	Died of cerebral infarction
2.5	Papillary RCC	−	Alive (13.2 years)
2.0	Clear cell carcinoma	−	Died of myocardial infarction (18.9 years)
2.9	Clear cell carcinoma	−	Alive (1.7 years)
3.5	Cyst-associated RCC	−	Alive (4.1 years)
3.5, 6.0 (Size of cyst)	*Clear cell carcinoma	−	Alive (1.8 years)
7.0 (including hematoma)	Papillary RCC	−	Alive (27.1 years)
2.5	Granular cell carcinoma	−	Died of cerebral bleeding (9.2 years)
2.3	Granular cell carcinoma	−	Died of uterine cancer (11 years)
2.4	*Clear cell carcinoma	−	Alive (16.6 years)
1.5	Granular cell carcinoma	−	Alive (9.7 years)
4.5	*Papillary RCC	−	Died of acute myocardial infarction (1.1 years)
0.3	*Papillary RCC	−	Died of gastric cancer
2.5	Oncocytoma Granular cell carcinoma	−	Alive (8.8 years)
1.0	*Papillary RCC	−	Alive (3.5 years)
1.7	Papillary RCC	−	Alive (13.6 years)
0.9	Oncocytoma	−	Died of perforation of peptic ulcer
4.5	*Papillary RCC	−	Died of perforation of jejunum (2.1 years)
1.8	Clear cell carcinoma	−	Died of sepsis
2.3	*Papillary RCC	−	Alive (3.6 years)
2.0	*Papillary RCC	−	Alive (13.2 years)
4.5	*Papillary RCC	−	Alive (17.4 years)
2.0	*Papillary RCC	−	Died of encapsulating peritoneal sclerosis
5.0 (including hematoma)	Clear cell carcinoma		
4.8	Granular cell carcinoma	+ (lymph node)	Died of RCC (0.8 year) (lung)
10.0 (including hematoma)	*Papillary RCC	+ (bone)	Died of RCC (0.7 year)
3.0	Spindle cell carcinoma		(lung, pleura, diaphragm, liver)
6.5	Papillary RCC	−	Alive (8.0 years)

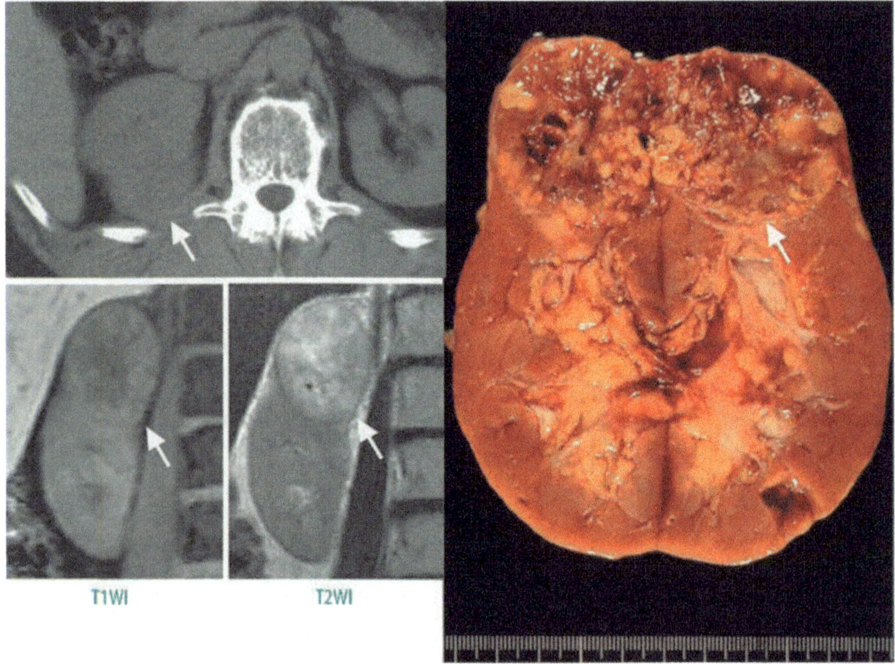

FIG. 73. Case 1. A 63-year-old man with chronic glomerulonephritis 2 months before the initiation of dialysis and with a high serum creatinine level (6.0 mg/dl). Clear cell carcinoma was detected before the initiation of dialysis. Clear cell carcinoma, pT1b,pNx,pMx,G2,INFα, v(−)

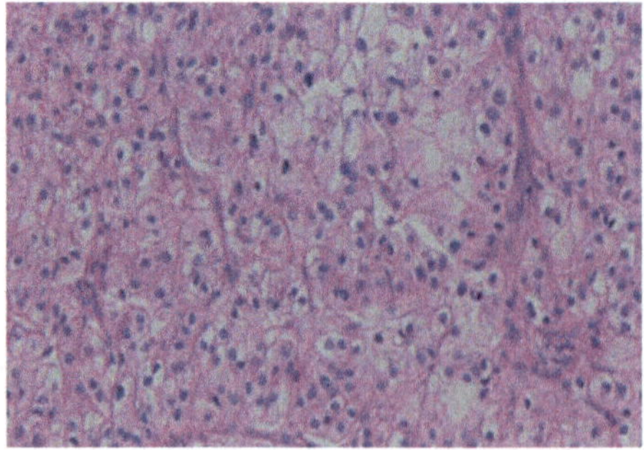

FIG. 74. Case 1. HE stain, ×200

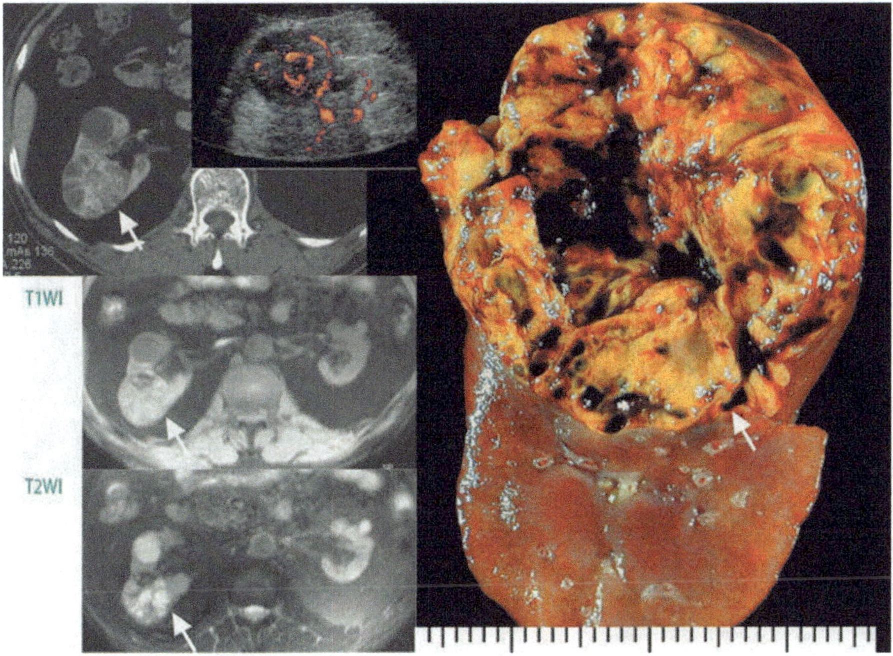

Fig. 75. Case 2. A 72-year-old man with chronic glomerulonephritis with a 3-day history of dialysis. Nephrectomy was performed because of clear cell carcinoma 3 days after the initiation of hemodialysis. Clear cell carcinoma, pT1b,pNx,pMx,G1>2,INFβ,v(−)

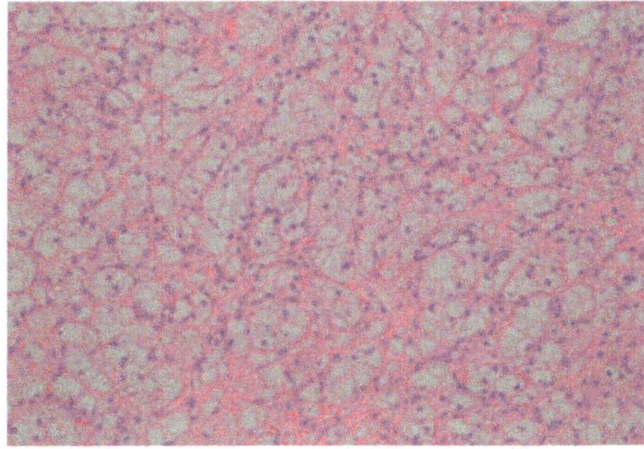

Fig. 76. Case 2. HE stain, ×100

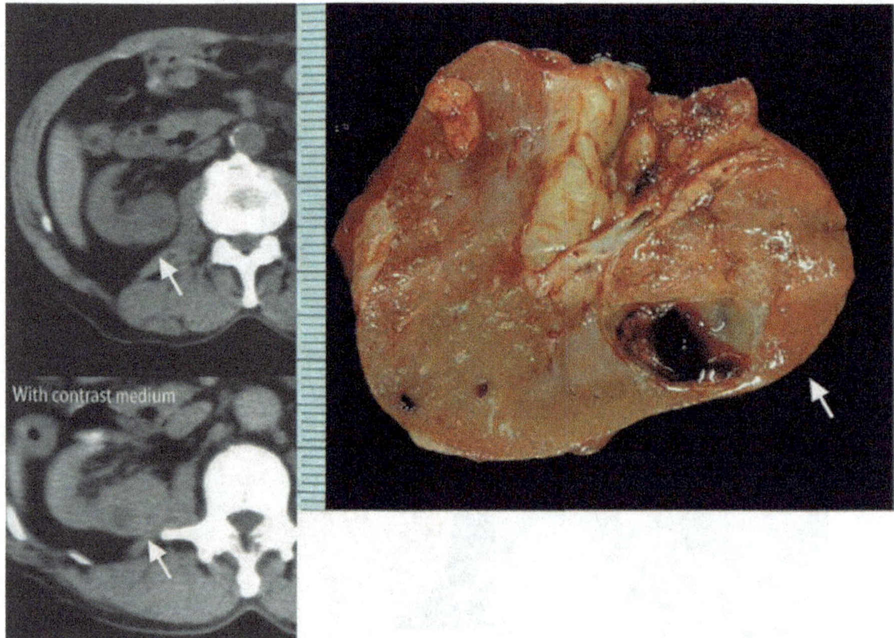

FIG. 77. Case 3. A 71-year-old man with possible chronic glomerulonephritis with a 2-month history of dialysis. This is a clear cell carcinoma in an elderly patient with a short history of dialysis. Clear cell carcinoma, pT1a,pNx,pMx,G1,INFα,v(−)

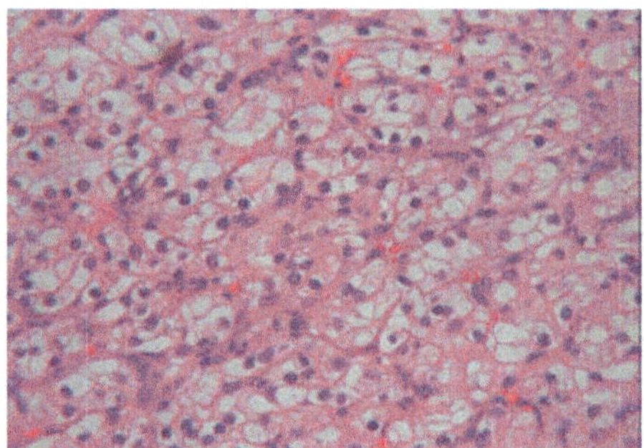

FIG. 78. Case 3. HE stain, ×400

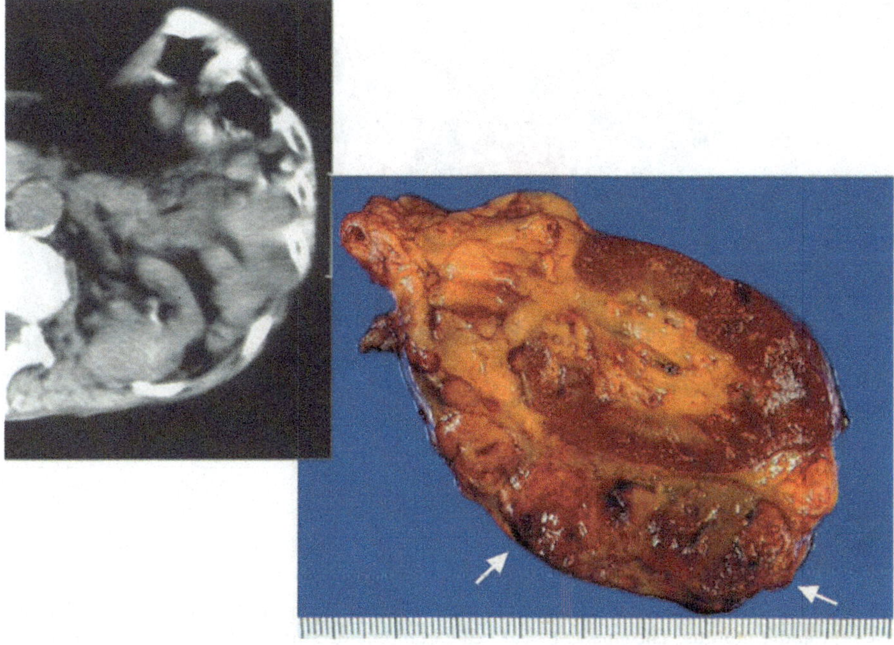

FIG. 79. Case 4. A 69-year-old man with possible chronic glomerulonephritis with a history of dialysis of 1 year and 2 months. This is a case of clear cell carcinoma with metastasis in a patient with a short history of dialysis. Clear cell carcinoma, pT3a,pN0,pM1,G3,INFβ,v(−)

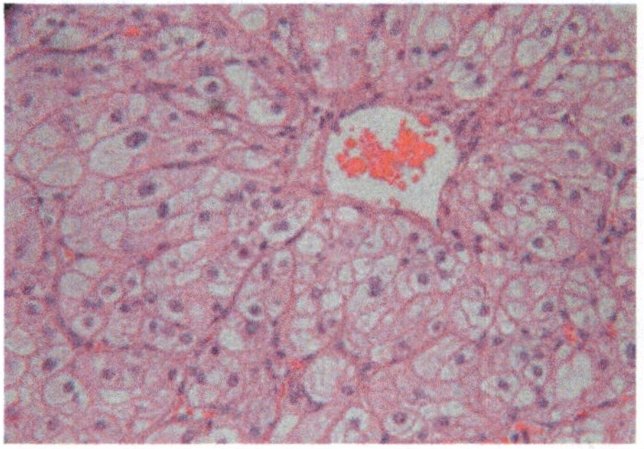

FIG. 80. Case 4. HE stain, ×400

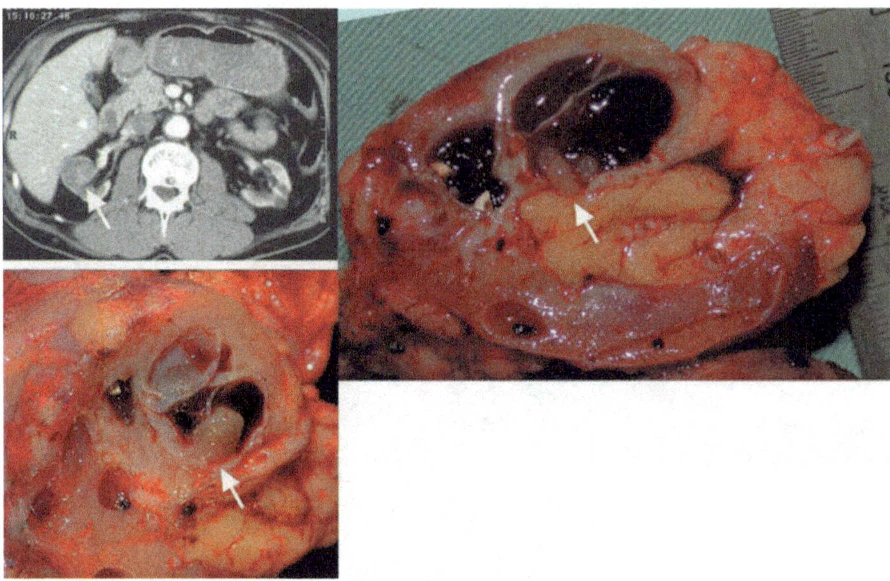

Fig. 81. Case 5. A 57-year-old man with chronic glomerulonephritis with a history of dialysis of 1 year and 4 months. The smallest clear cell carcinoma of 5 mm in diameter could be diagnosed. Clear cell carcinoma, pT1a,pNx,pMx,G2,INFα,v(−)

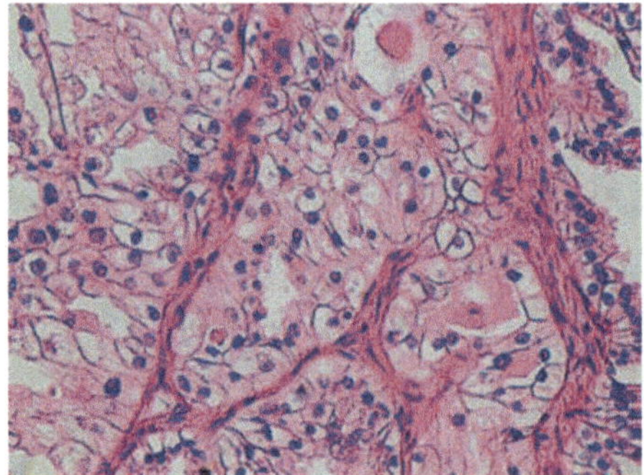

Fig. 82. Case 5. HE stain, ×400

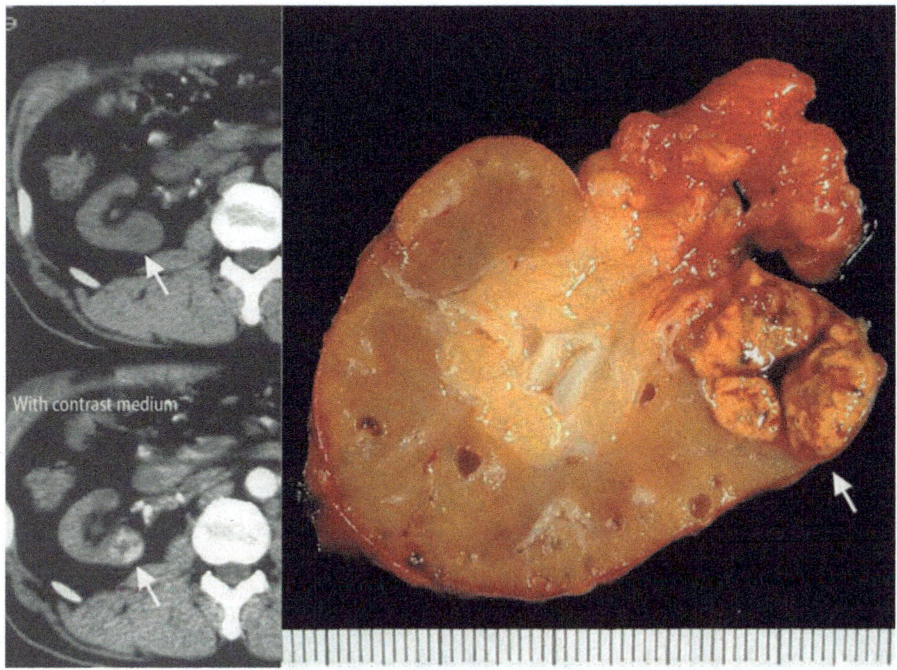

Fig. 83. Case 6. A 43-year-old man with chronic glomerulonephritis with a history of dialysis of 2 years and 2 months. Clear cell carcinoma was detected by CT screening. Clear cell carcinoma, pT1a,pNx,pMx,G1,INFα,v(−)

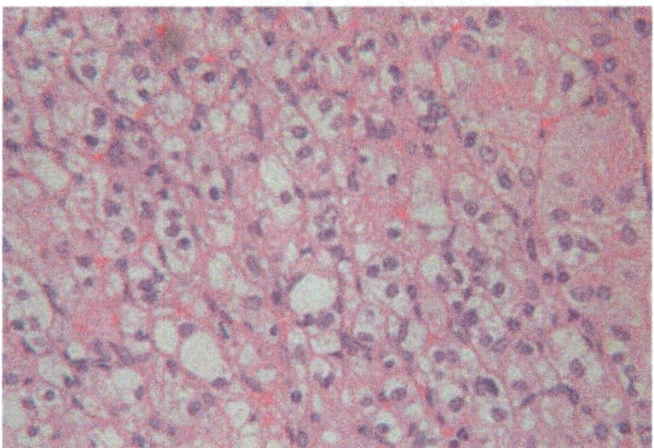

Fig. 84. Case 6. HE stain, ×400

Case 7. A 63-year-old woman with diabetic nephropathy and with a history of dialysis of 2 years and 7 months. This was a clear cell carcinoma observed in an elderly patient with a short history of dialysis (Figs. 85 and 86). The renal parenchyma appeared to be thickened in the area of the left kidney, as indicated by the arrow. However, it was rare that the renal parenchyma remained only in this area in end-stage renal failure, and the finding was considered to be abnormal. Contrast enhance-

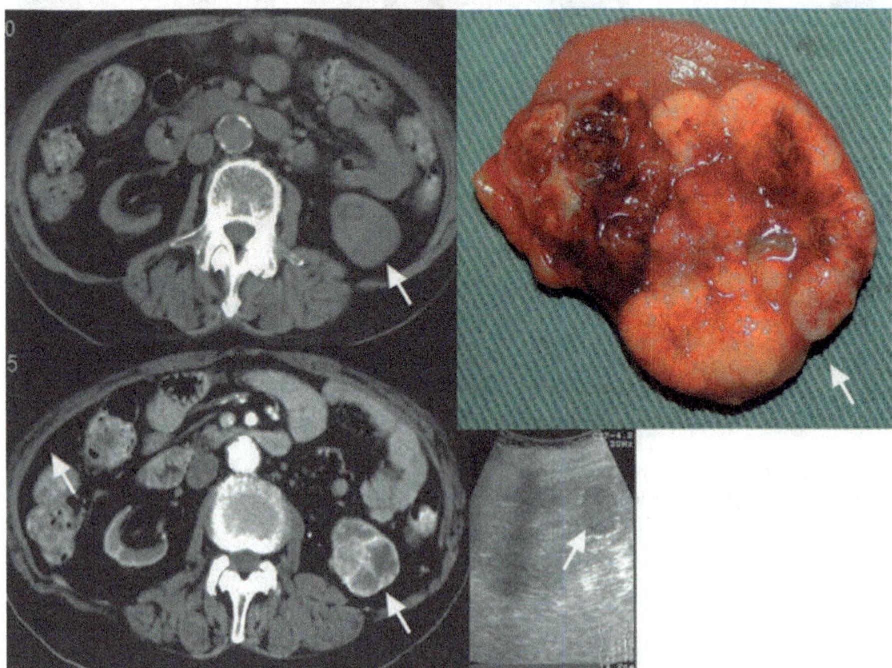

FIG. 85. Case 7. A 63-year-old woman with diabetic nephropathy with a history of dialysis of 2 years and 7 months. This is a case of clear cell carcinoma in an elderly patient with a short history of dialysis. Clear cell carcinoma, pT1a,pNx,pMx,G2>1,INFα,v(−) (CT in the lower panel: Reproduced from [6], by permission of Oxford University Press)

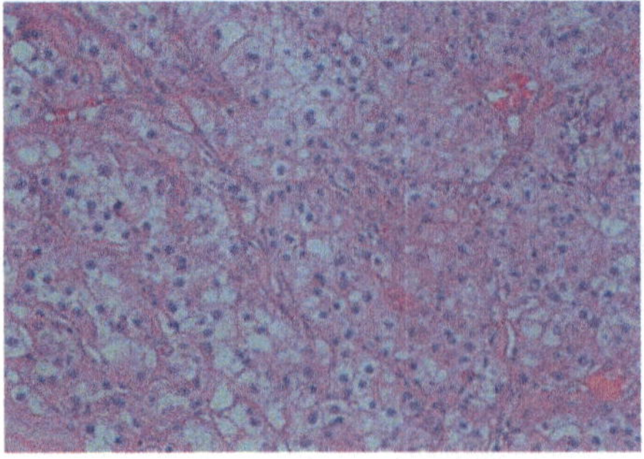

FIG. 86. Case 7. HE stain, ×200

ment was observed by dynamic CT, and a diagnosis of renal cell carcinoma was made.

Case 8. A 64-year-old woman with diabetic nephropathy and with a history of dialysis of 2 years and 11 months. This was a clear cell carcinoma observed in an elderly patient with a short history of dialysis (Figs. 87 and 88). Protrusion of the mass from the renal margin suggested renal cell carcinoma, and a diagnosis of hypervascular tumor was made by dynamic CT.

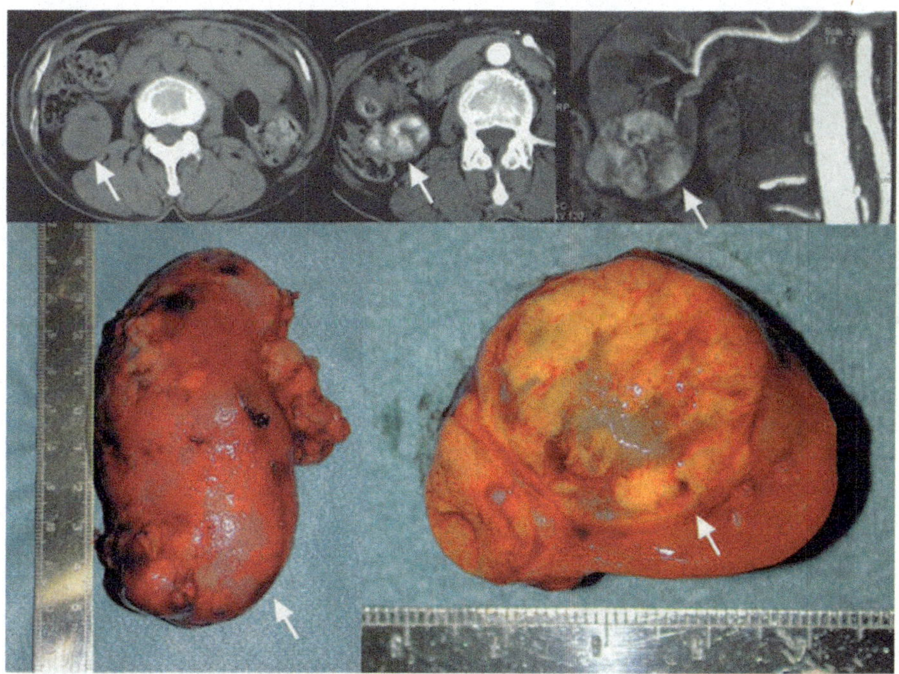

FIG. 87. Case 8. A 64-year-old woman with diabetic nephropathy with a history of dialysis of 2 years and 11 months. This is a case of clear cell carcinoma in an elderly patient with a short history of dialysis. Clear cell carcinoma, pT1a,pNx,pMx,G2>1,INFα,v(−)

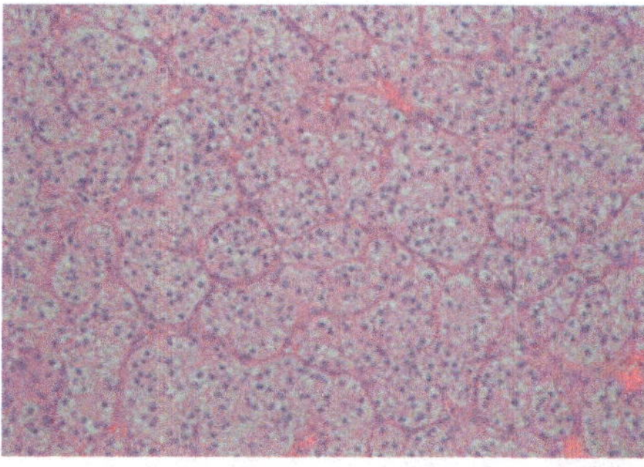

FIG. 88. Case 8. HE stain, ×100

Case 9. A 65-year-old man with diabetic nephropathy and with a 4-year history of continuous ambulatory peritoneal dialysis (CAPD). A granular cell carcinoma was confirmed by autopsy (Figs. 89 and 90). No protrusion was observed in the left kidney by CT performed before death.

Case 10. A 44-year-old man with chronic glomerulonephritis and with a history of dialysis of 5 years and 5 months. This was a case of metachronous bilateral renal cell carcinoma, also with a lesion in the opposite kidney (Figs. 91 and 92). An opposite lesion was found in Case 28. Hematuria was noted, and CT revealed a hypervascular tumor.

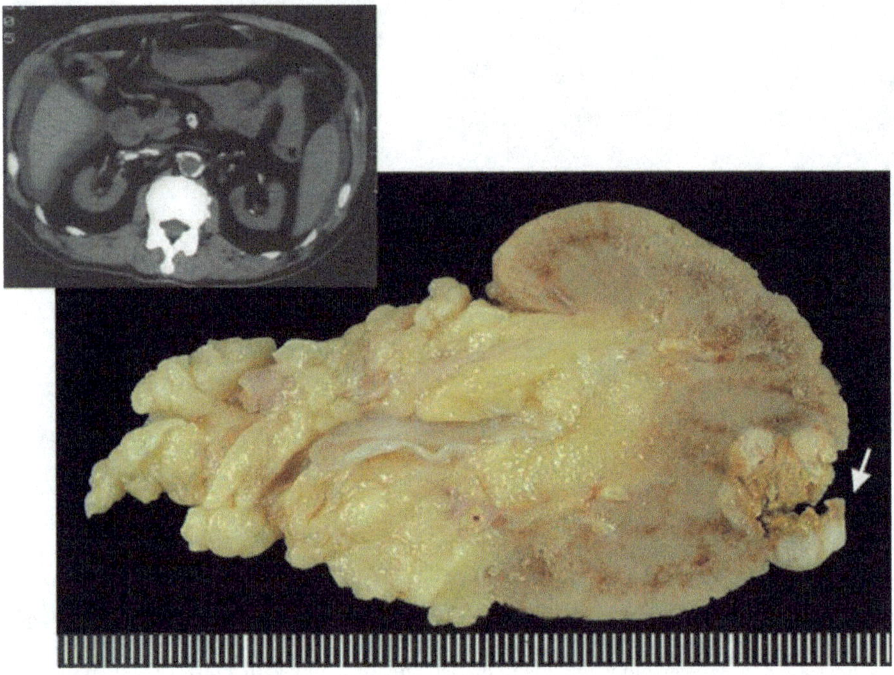

Fig. 89. Case 9. A 65-year-old man with diabetic nephropathy with a 4-year history of CAPD. Granular cell carcinoma was found at autopsy, and was not suspected from CT before death. Granular cell carcinoma, pT1a,pN0,pM0,G1,INFα,v(−)

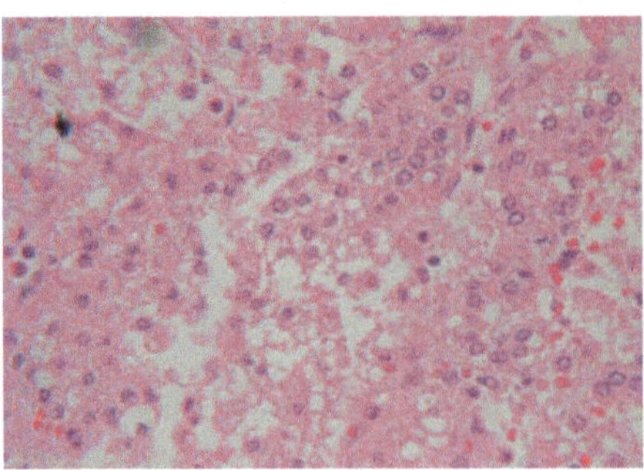

Fig. 90. Case 9. HE stain, ×400

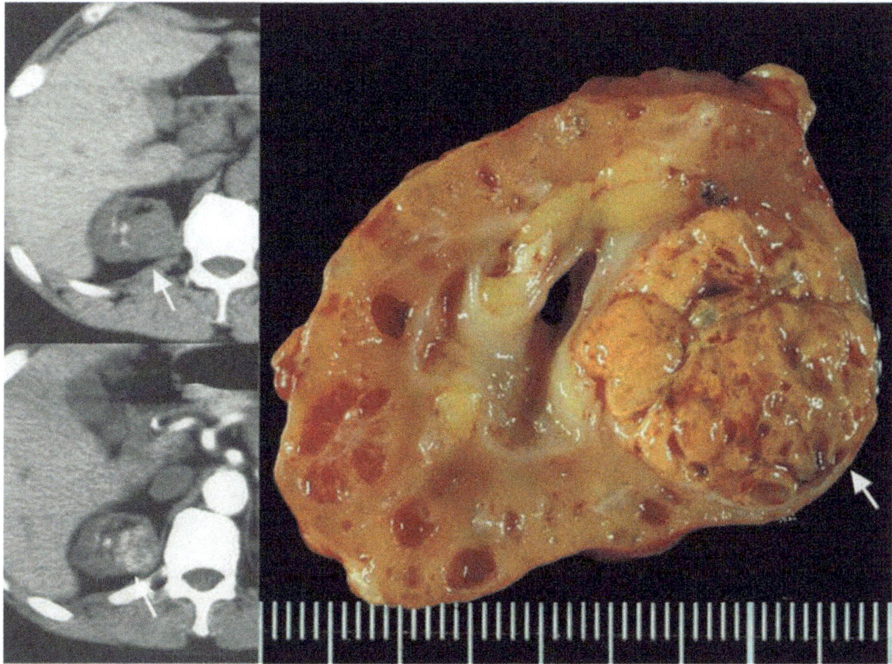

FIG. 91. Case 10. A 44-year-old man with chronic glomerulonephritis with a history of dialysis of 5 years and 5 months. This is a case of metachronous bilateral renal cell carcinoma. The lesion in the opposite kidney is Case 28. Papillary renal cell carcinoma, pT1a,pNx,pMx,G1>>2, INFα,v(−)

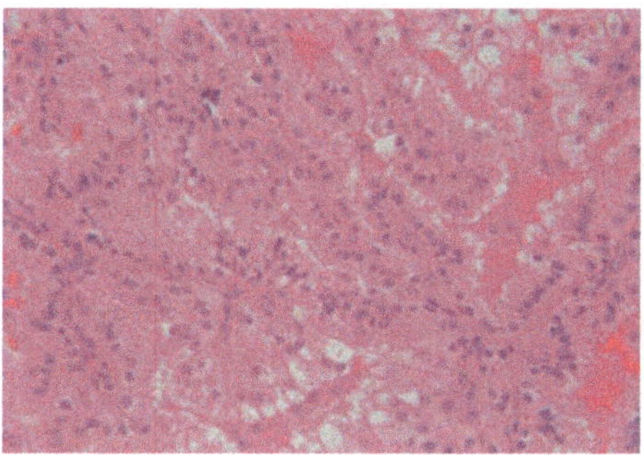

FIG. 92. Case 10. HE stain, ×200

Case 11. A 28-year-old man with chronic glomerulonephritis and with a history of dialysis of 5 years and 8 months. This was an early case of clear cell carcinoma detected by screening, and the patient underwent bilateral nephrectomy (Figs. 93 and 94). A tumor with a calcified margin was observed. No cyst appeared to be present in the renal parenchyma or other areas by CT scan, but small cysts were noted in the resected kidneys.

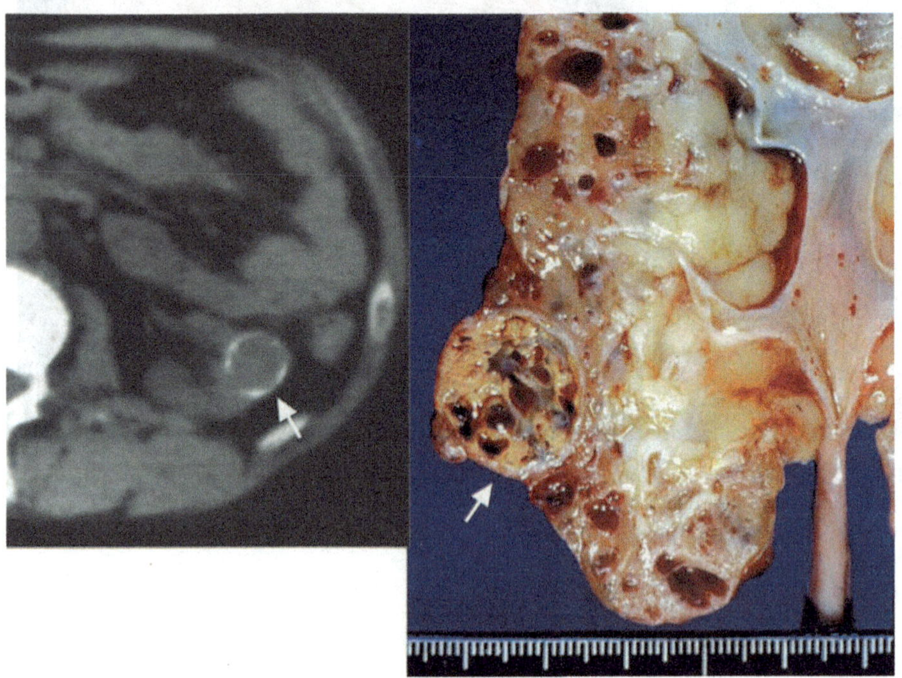

FIG. 93. Case 11. A 28-year-old man with chronic glomerulonephritis with a history of dialysis of 5 years and 8 months. This is an early case in which clear cell carcinoma was detected by screening, and bilateral nephrectomy was performed. Clear cell carcinoma, pT1a, pNx,pMx,G1,INFα,v(−)

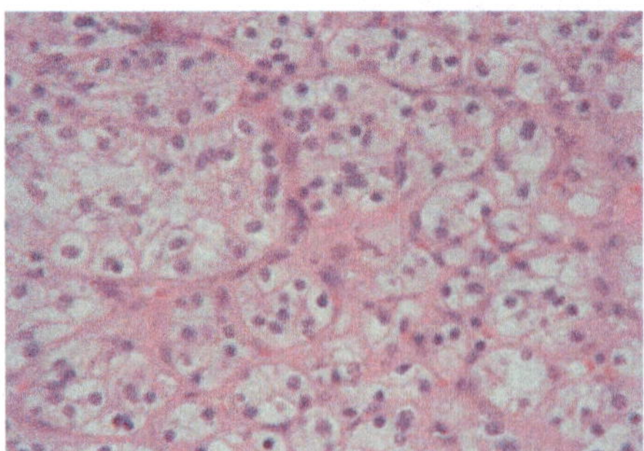

FIG. 94. Case 11. HE stain, ×400

Case 12. A 73-year-old man with chronic glomerulonephritis and with a history of dialysis of 6 years. A clear cell carcinoma was detected by CT screening (Figs. 95 and 96). A T1WI mass with similar signal intensity to that of the renal parenchyma was observed.

Case 13. A 34-year-old man with a 6-year history of dialysis, with chronic glomerulonephritis 9 months after renal transplantation. Cystic renal cell carcinoma was present in the area that showed no regression of cysts after renal transplantation [72]

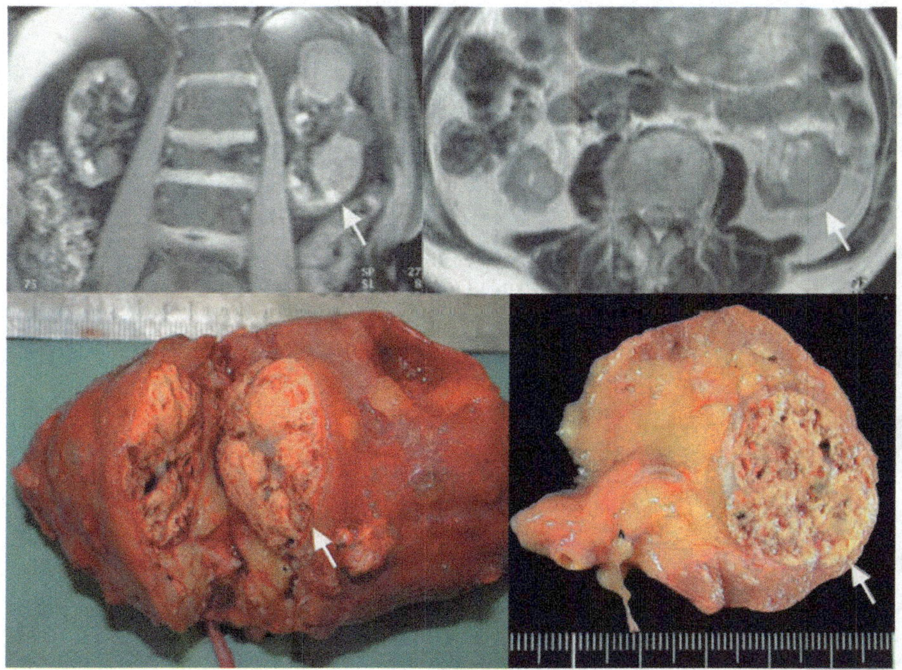

FIG. 95. Case 12. A 73-year-old man with chronic glomerulonephritis and with a 6-year history of dialysis. The clear cell carcinoma was detected by CT screening. Clear cell carcinoma, pT1a,pNx,pMx,G2>1,INFα,v(−)

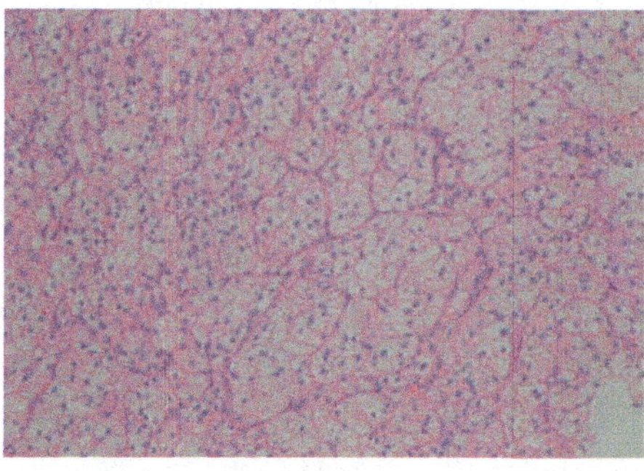

FIG. 96. Case 12. HE stain, ×100

(Figs. 97 and 98). Since the cyst size in this area alone did not change even 9 months after renal transplantation, nephrectomy was performed, and cystic renal cell carcinoma was confirmed. Note the yellow color of the surface of the resected kidney. After renal transplantation, few cysts in the right kidney persisted, but those in the left kidney mostly disappeared except in the region of the renal cell carcinoma.

Case 14. A 30-year-old woman with a 7-month history of dialysis, and with chronic glomerulonephritis 5 years and 8 months after renal transplantation. Renal cell

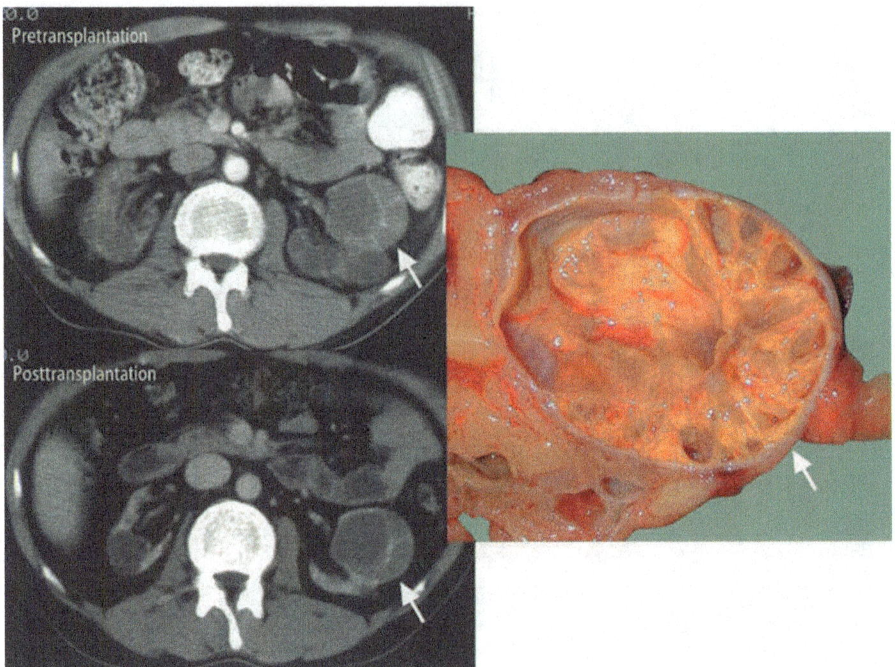

FIG. 97. Case 13. A 34-year-old man with chronic glomerulonephritis 9 months after renal transplantation, and with a 6-year history of dialysis. The cystic renal cell carcinoma was found in an area that did not show cyst regression after renal transplantation. Cystic renal cell carcinoma, pT1a,pNx,pMx,G1,INFα,v(−) (Reproduced from [72])

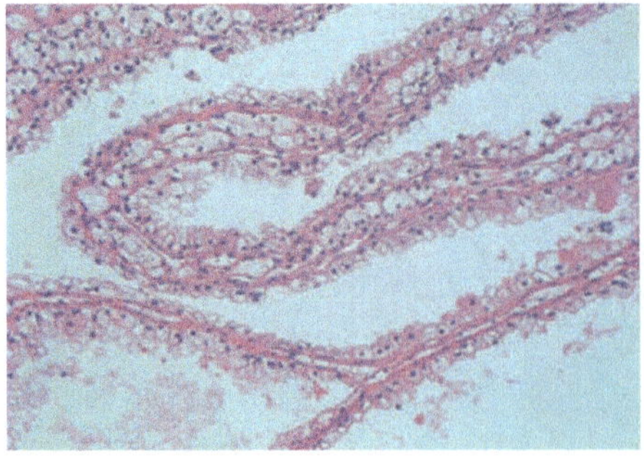

FIG. 98. Case 13. HE stain, ×100 (Reproduced from [72])

carcinoma occurred at 2 sites in the right kidney after renal transplantation [51] (Figs. 99 and 100). Masses in the upper (yellow arrows) and lower (white arrows) poles of the kidney enlarged into a tumor of the cyst wall and a solid (hypervascular) tumor, respectively, 5 years and 8 months after renal transplantation.

Case 15. A 24-year-old man with rapidly progressive glomerulonephritis and with a history of dialysis of 6 years and 11 months. This is the first clinical case in the world in which acquired cystic disease of the kidney was complicated by renal cell

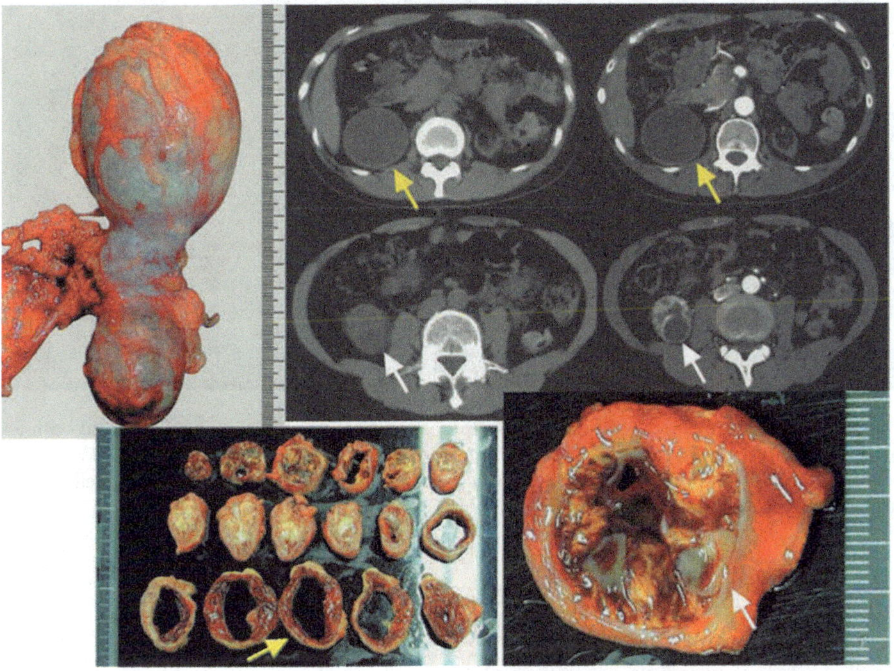

FIG. 99. Case 14. A 30-year-old woman with chronic glomerulonephritis 5 years and 8 months after renal transplantation, and with a 7-month history of dialysis. This is a case in which renal cell carcinoma occurred at two sites in the right kidney after renal transplantation. Clear cell carcinoma, pT1a,pNx,pMx,G1>2,INFα,v(−)

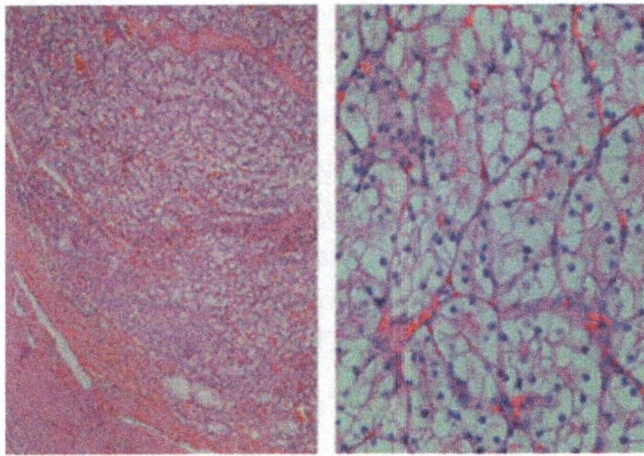

FIG. 100. Case 14. HE stain: *left*, ×40; *right*, ×200

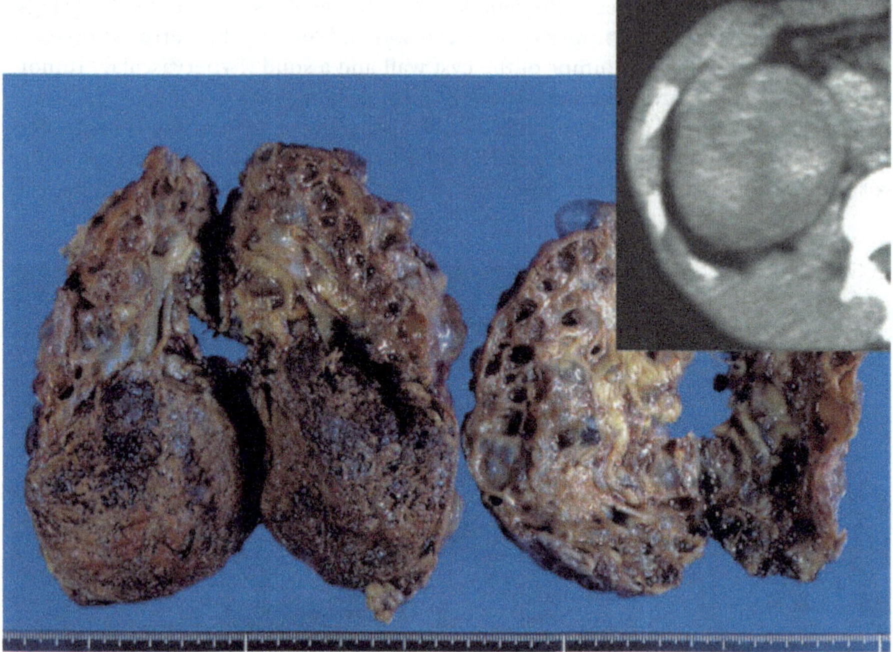

Fig. 101. Case 15. A 24-year-old man with rapidly progressive glomerulonephritis and with a history of dialysis of 6 years and 11 months. This was the world's first clinical case. Papillary renal cell carcinoma occurred in the wall of a very large hematoma. Papillary renal cell carcinoma, pT1a,pNx,pMx,G1,INFα,v(−)

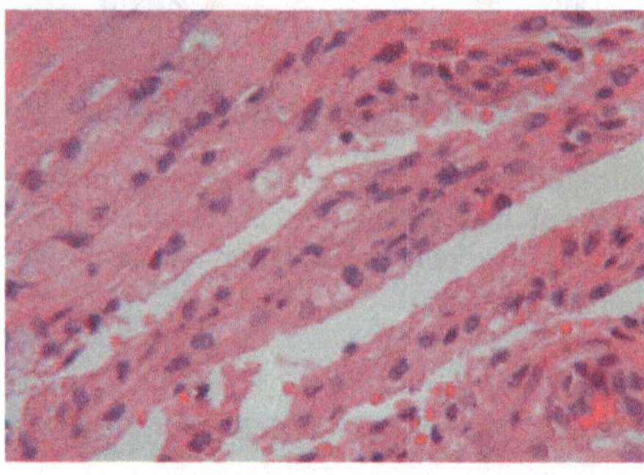

Fig. 102. Case 15. HE stain, ×400

carcinoma. A papillary renal cell carcinoma was observed in the wall of a very large hematoma (Figs. 101 and 102). This was an early case in which plain CT delineated a mass suggestive of a very large hematoma.

Case 16. A 31-year-old man with chronic glomerulonephritis and with a history of dialysis of 7 years and 8 months. Renal cell carcinoma was detected at an unexpected site (Figs. 103 and 104). In this patient, who had a long history of dialysis, the mass

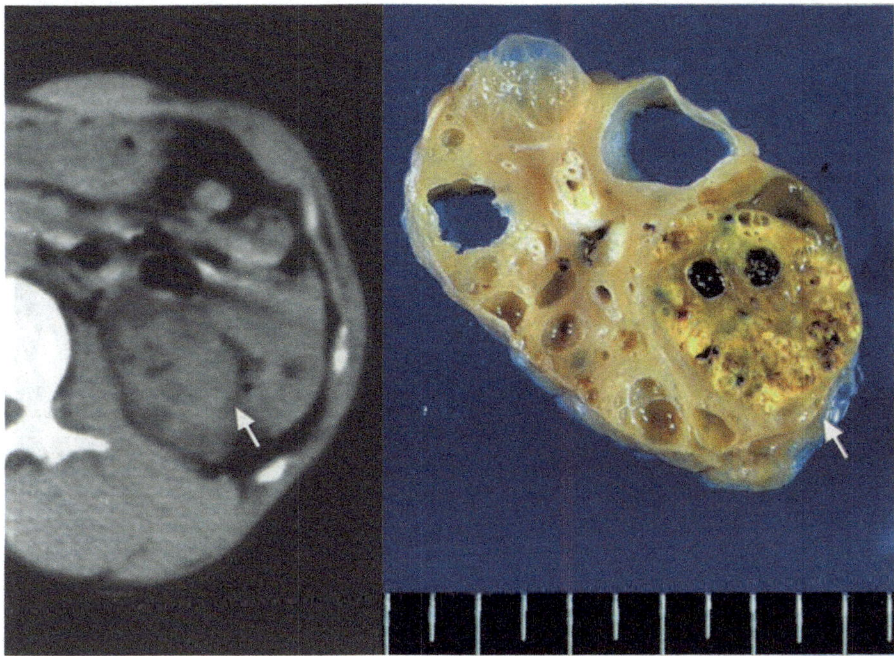

FIG. 103. Case 16. A 31-year-old man with chronic glomerulonephritis and with a history of dialysis of 7 years and 8 months. Renal cell carcinoma was detected at an unexpected site not protruding from the renal margin. Granular cell carcinoma, pT1a,pNx,pMx,G1,INFα,v(−) (Reproduced from [34], with permission from Elsevier Inc.)

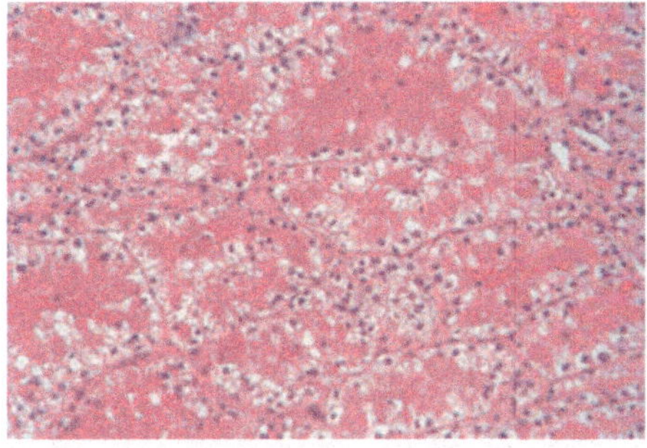

FIG. 104. Case 16. HE stain, ×100

did not protrude from the renal margin, and small acquired renal cysts were observed in large numbers in areas other than the renal cell carcinoma.

Case 17. A 28-year-old woman with chronic glomerulonephritis and with a history of dialysis of 8 years. This was an early case, detected by screening, in which renal cell carcinoma was complicated by multiple cancers (uterine cancer) (Figs. 105 and 106). The mass appeared to be residual renal parenchyma or a protrusion from the renal margin.

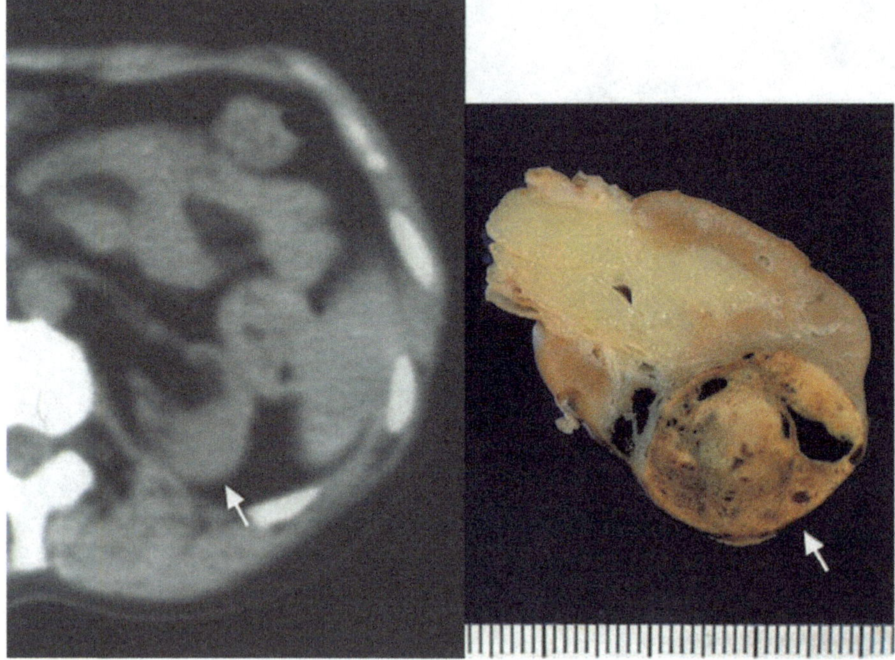

Fig. 105. Case 17. A 28-year-old woman with chronic glomerulonephritis and with an 8-year history of dialysis. An early screened case with multiple cancers (uterine cancer). Granular cell carcinoma, pT1a,pNx,pMx,G1,INFα,v(−) (Reproduced from [2], with permission from Dustri-Verlag Dr. Karl Feistle)

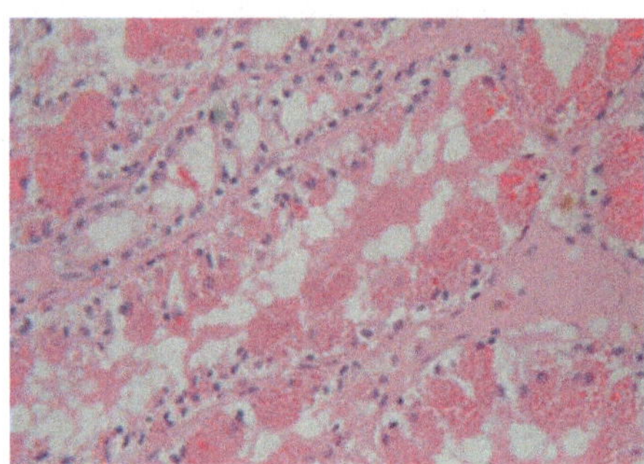

Fig. 106. Case 17. HE stain, ×200

Case 18. A 39-year-old man with an 8-month history of dialysis, and with chronic glomerulonephritis 8 years and 4 months after renal transplantation. Renal cell carcinoma was detected 7 years and 4 months after renal transplantation [52], but it may have occurred preoperatively (Figs. 107 and 108). Among the cysts that persisted in the native kidney after renal transplantation, the one indicated by the arrows showed intense contrast enhancement.

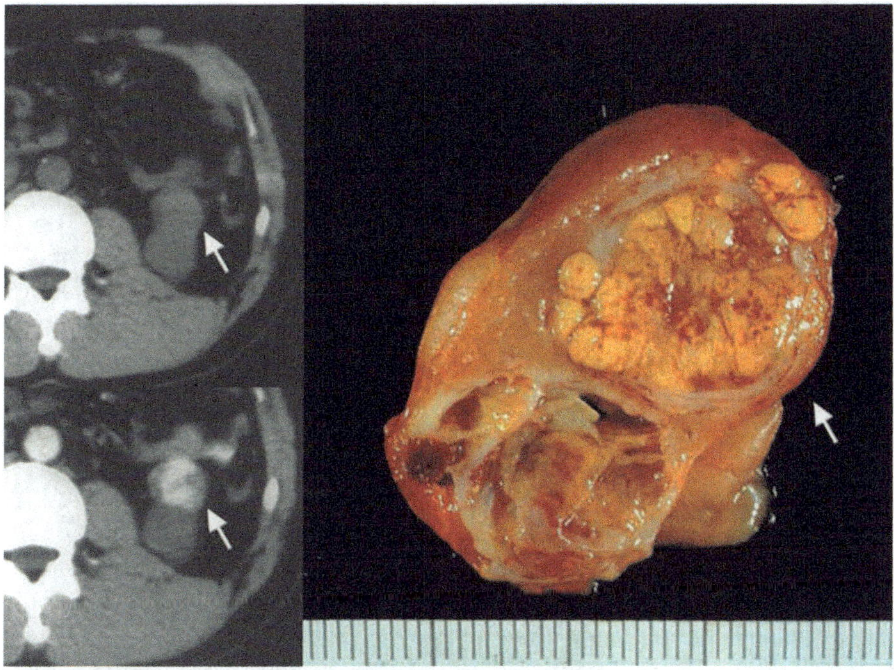

FIG. 107. Case 18. A 39-year-old man with chronic glomerulonephritis 8 years and 4 months after renal transplantation, and with an 8-month history of dialysis before transplantation. The renal cell carcinoma may have been present from before the renal transplantation, but was only detected 8 years and 4 months after surgery. Clear cell carcinoma, pT1a,pNx,pMx,G1, INFα,v(−)

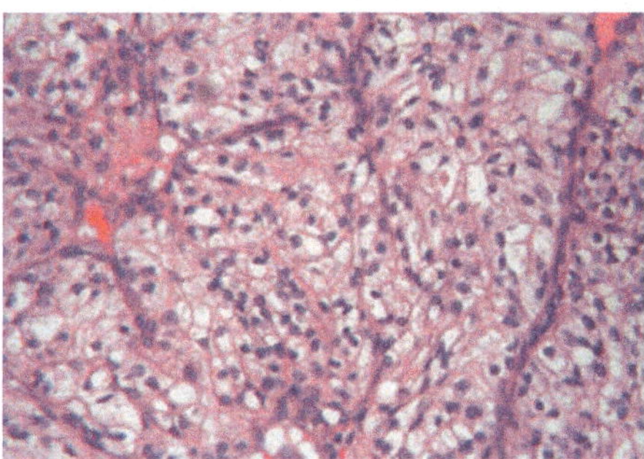

FIG. 108. Case 18. HE stain, ×200

Case 19. A 38-year-old woman with toxemia of pregnancy and a history of dialysis of 8 years and 11 months. This is a case of a clear cell carcinoma observed in a dialysis patient (Figs. 109 and 110). During the follow-up, a mass developed in the interior of the kidney and showed contrast enhancement.

Case 20. A 62-year-old man with diabetic nephropathy and with a history of dialysis (CAPD) of 9 years and 6 months. An example of a papillary renal cell carcinoma

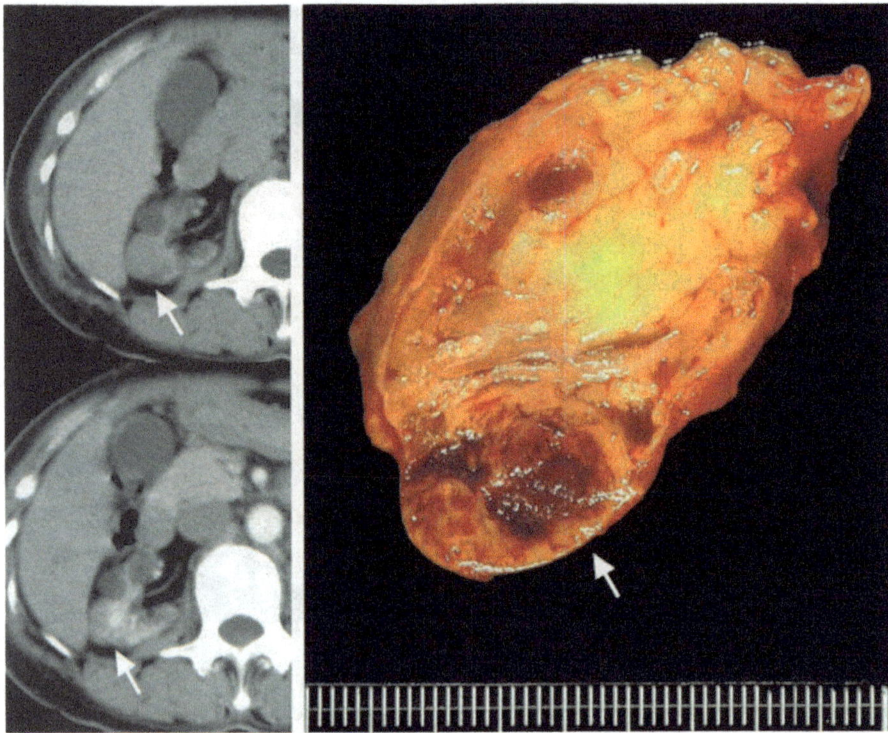

FIG. 109. Case 19. A 38-year-old woman with a history of dialysis of 8 years and 11 months due to toxemia of pregnancy. This is a case of clear cell carcinoma in a dialysis patient. Granular cell carcinoma, pT1a,pNx,pMx,G1>2,INFα,v(−)

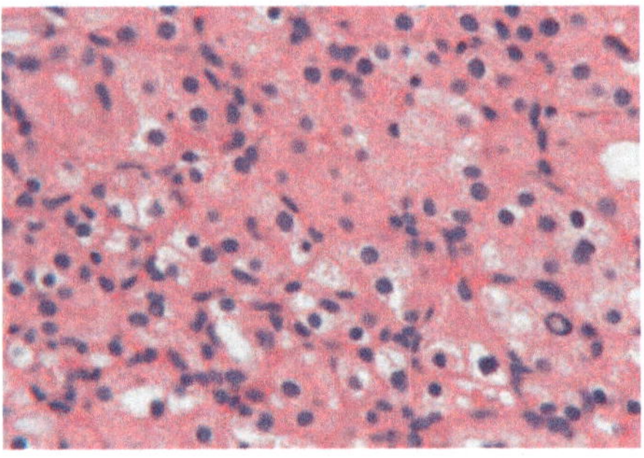

FIG. 110. Case 19. HE stain, ×400

observed in the left kidney of a patient on long-term CAPD (Figs. 111 and 112). The tumor had partially invaded the left renal vein (yellow arrows). A renal cell carcinoma extended from the hilum to the lower pole of the left kidney (white arrows). The tumor was hypovascular with weak contrast enhancement, and did not protrude from the renal margin.

Case 21. A 47-year-old man with chronic glomerulonephritis and with a history of dialysis of 10 years and 7 months. The patient died from gastric cancer, but an autopsy

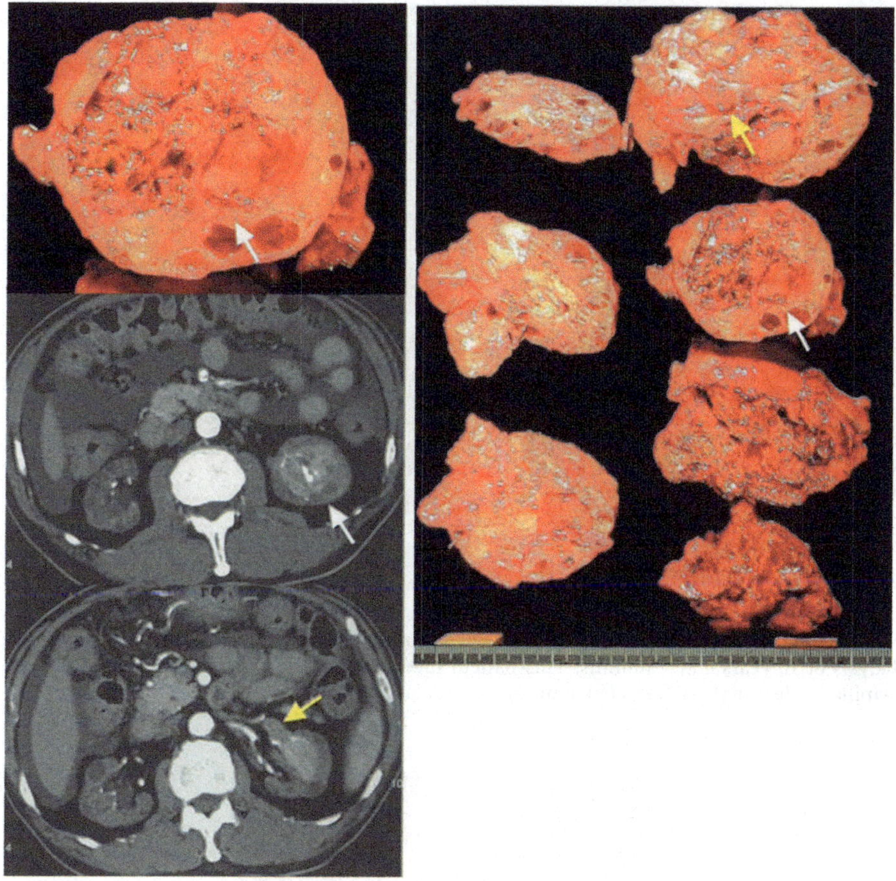

FIG. 111. Case 20. A 62-year-old man with diabetic nephropathy with a history of CAPD of 9 years and 6 months. This is a case of papillary renal cell carcinoma in a patient receiving CAPD. There was venous infiltration. Papillary renal cell carcinoma, pT3b,pNx,pMx,G2,INFα,v(+)

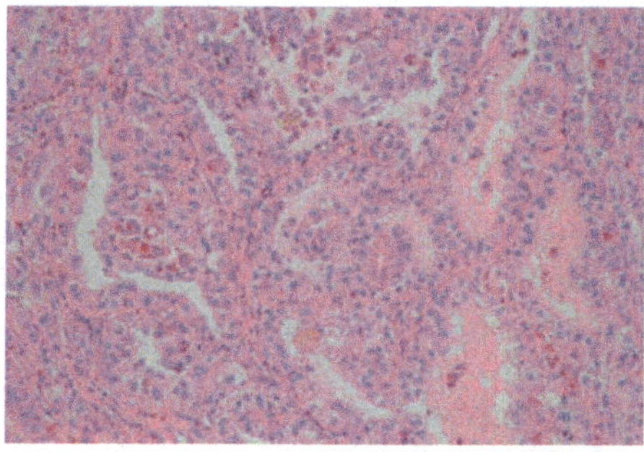

FIG. 112. Case 20. HE stain, ×200

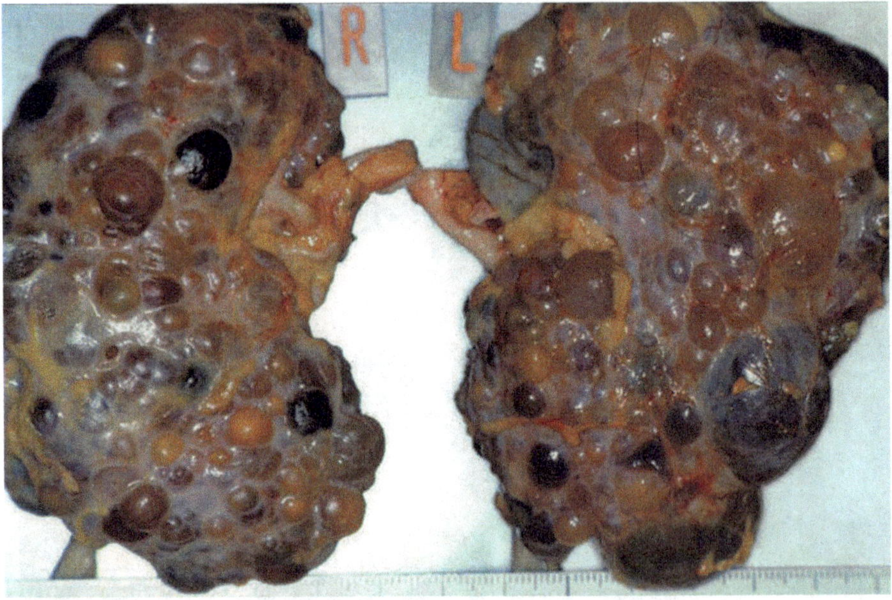

FIG. 113. Case 21. A 47-year-old man with chronic glomerulonephritis and with a history of dialysis of 10 years and 7 months. This patient died from gastric cancer, and a renal tumor (papillary adenoma) was detected at autopsy. Papillary renal adenoma

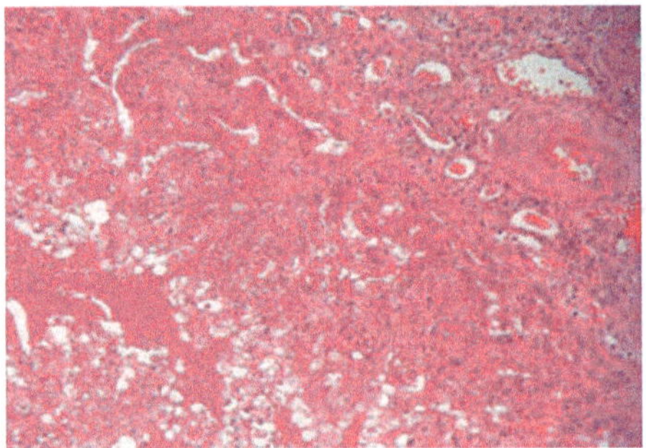

FIG. 114. Case 21. HE stain, ×100

revealed a renal tumor (papillary adenoma) (Figs. 113 and 114). CT performed before death indicated only acquired cystic disease of the kidney with no mass.

Case 22. A 55-year-old woman with chronic glomerulonephritis and with a history of dialysis of 11 years and 3 months. The patient developed renal cell carcinoma and oncocytoma (Figs. 115 and 116). A mass that showed contrast enhancement was detected by periodic CT screening, and surgery was performed, resulting in the detection of an oncocytoma 2.5 cm in diameter.

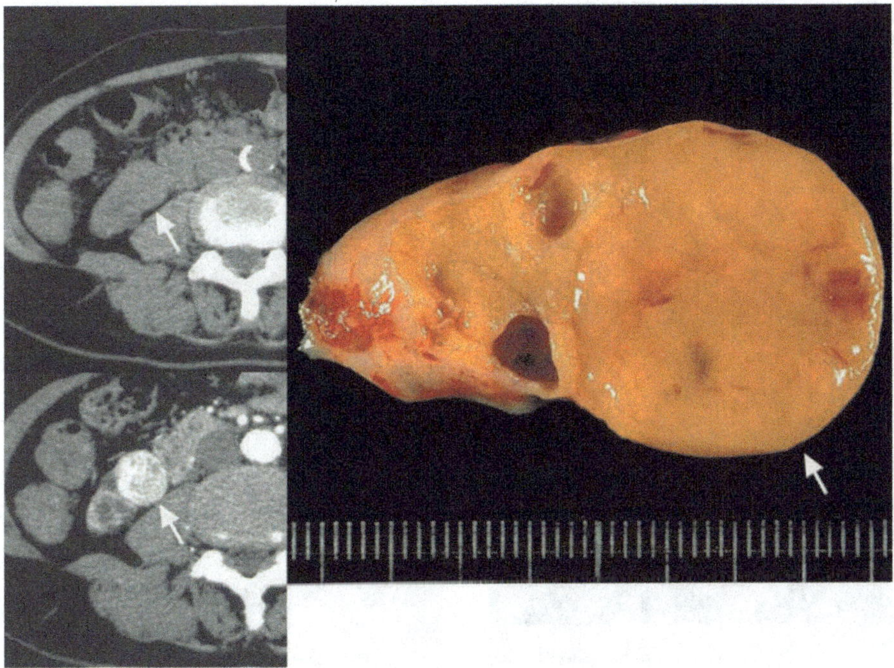

Fig. 115. Case 22. A 55-year-old woman with chronic glomerulonephritis and with a history of dialysis of 11 years and 3 months. This is a case of oncocytoma

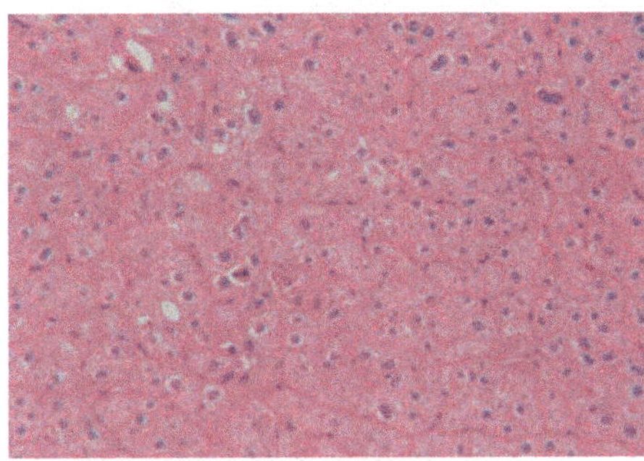

Fig. 116. Case 22. HE stain, ×200

Case 23. A 41-year-old man with chronic glomerulonephritis and with a history of dialysis of 11 years and 3 months. Nephrectomy was performed because of retroperitoneal bleeding, and papillary renal cell carcinoma 1 cm in diameter in the cyst wall was detected (Figs. 117 and 118).

Case 24. A 41-year-old man with an 11-year history of dialysis, and with chronic glomerulonephritis 5 months after renal transplantation. The patient had been suspected to have renal cell carcinoma before renal transplantation, and surgery was

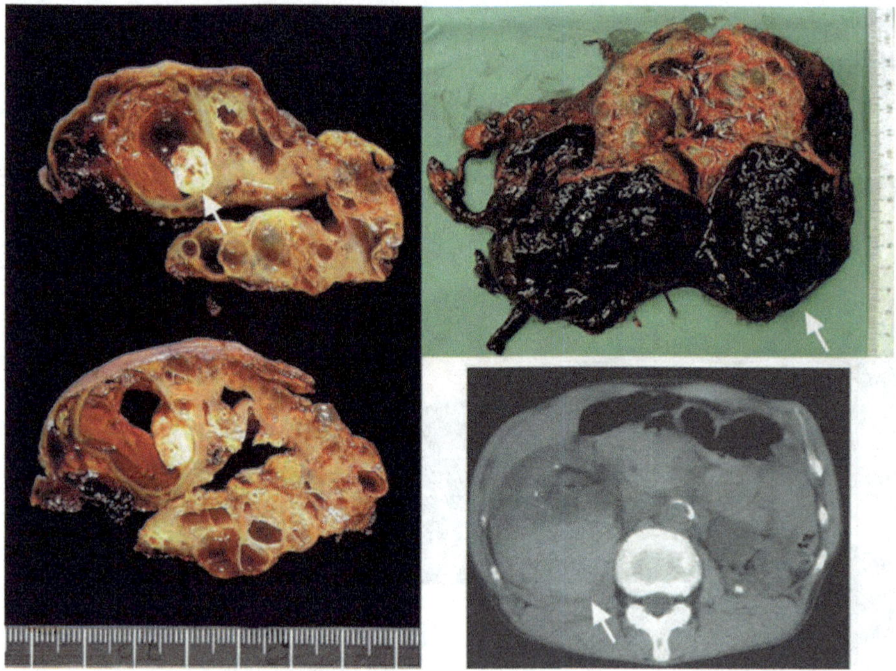

FIG. 117. Case 23. A 41-year-old man with chronic glomerulonephritis and with a history of dialysis of 11 years and 3 months. Nephrectomy was performed because of retroperitoneal bleeding, and papillary renal cell carcinoma was found in the resected kidney. Papillary renal cell carcinoma, pT1a,pNx,pMx,G2,INFα,v(−)

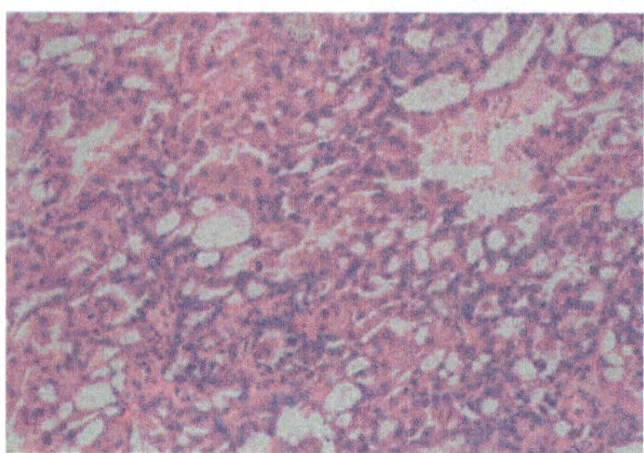

FIG. 118. Case 23. HE stain, ×200

performed because no postoperative regression was observed at the site of the tumor [118] (Figs. 119 and 120). Dynamic CT was performed before renal transplantation, but little contrast enhancement was observed (white arrows), and the diagnosis of renal cell carcinoma was uncertain. However, diagnosis became possible after renal transplantation because cysts regressed except in the suspected area. At this time, contrast enhancement (yellow arrows) was confirmed on enhanced MRI using gadolinium-diethylenetriaminopentoacetic acid (Gd-DTPA).

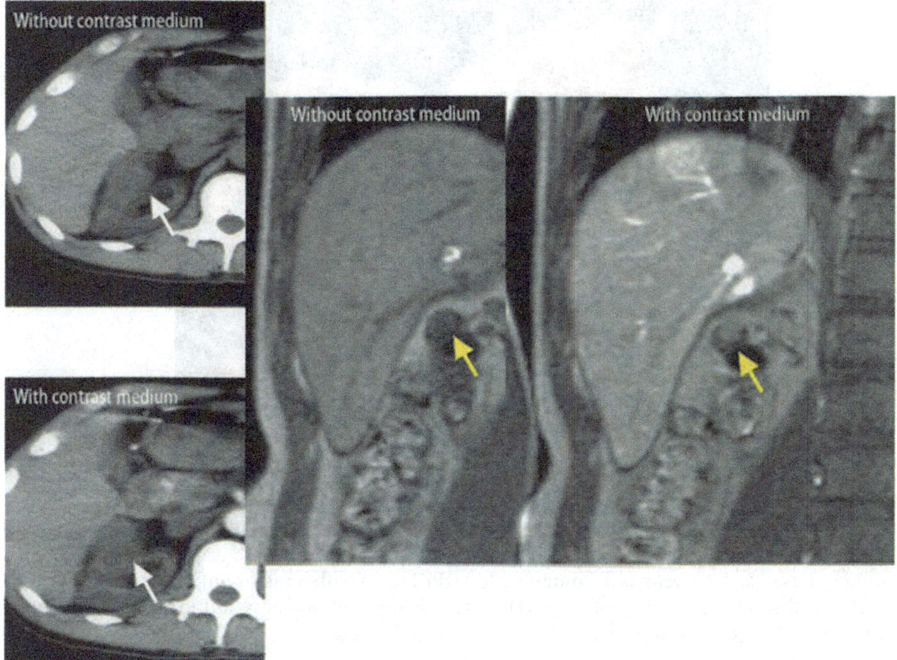

FIG. 119. Case 24. A 41-year-old man with chronic glomerulonephritis 5 months after renal transplantation, and with an 11-year history of dialysis. Renal cell carcinoma was suspected before renal transplantation, and nephrectomy was performed because there was no regression at the suspected site after renal transplantation. Papillary renal cell carcinoma, pT1a,pNx,pMx, G2,INFα,v(−) (Reproduced from [118], with permission from Elsevier Inc.)

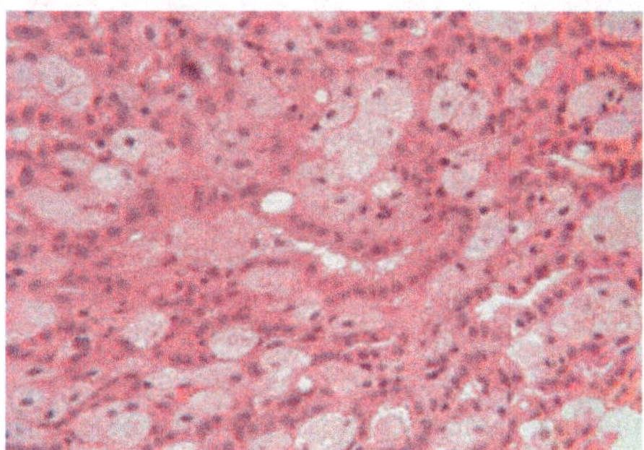

FIG. 120. Case 24. HE stain, ×200

Case 25. A 64-year-old woman with autosomal dominant polycystic kidney disease (ADPKD) and with a history of dialysis of 12 years and 2 months. At autopsy, the autosomal dominant polycystic kidney disease was found to be complicated by oncocytoma (Figs. 121 and 122). The diagnosis was impossible by imaging studies before death.

Case 26. A 64-year-old man with possible chronic glomerulonephritis and with a history of dialysis of 13 years. The patient had papillary renal cell carcinoma and

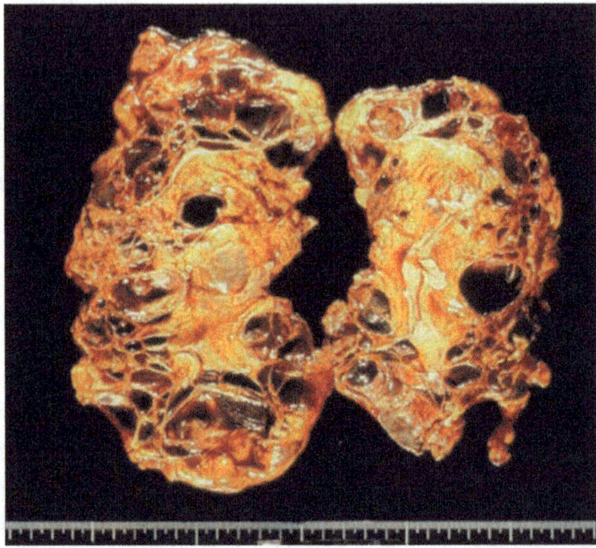

FIG. 121. Case 25. A 64-year-old woman with ADPKD and with a history of dialysis of 12 years and 2 months. This is a case of ADPKD in which oncocytoma was found at autopsy (not observed in the cross section). Oncocytoma 9 mm in diameter

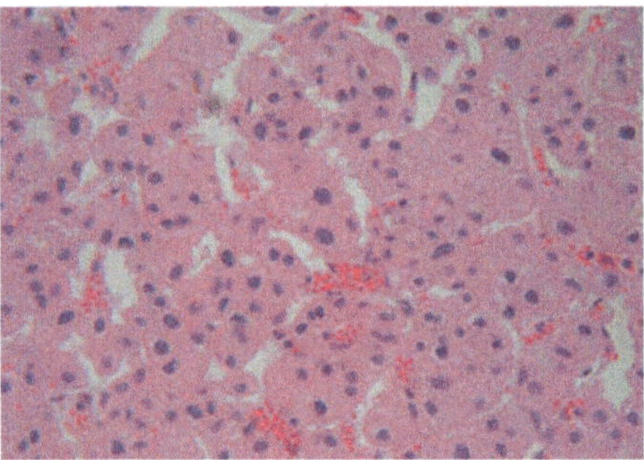

FIG. 122. Case 25. HE stain, ×400

multiple cancers (Figs. 123 and 124), and underwent nephrectomy, thyroidectomy, and parathyroidectomy due to thyroid cancer and secondary hyperparathyroidism. A hypovascular tumor was detected in the lower pole of the right kidney by dynamic CT.

Case 27. A 68-year-old man with chronic glomerulonephritis and with a history of dialysis of 13 years and 6 months. Renal cell carcinoma was suspected before death, and clear cell carcinoma was confirmed at autopsy (Figs. 125 and 126). Although CT and MRI suggested renal cell carcinoma, surgery could not be performed because of the patient's poor general condition.

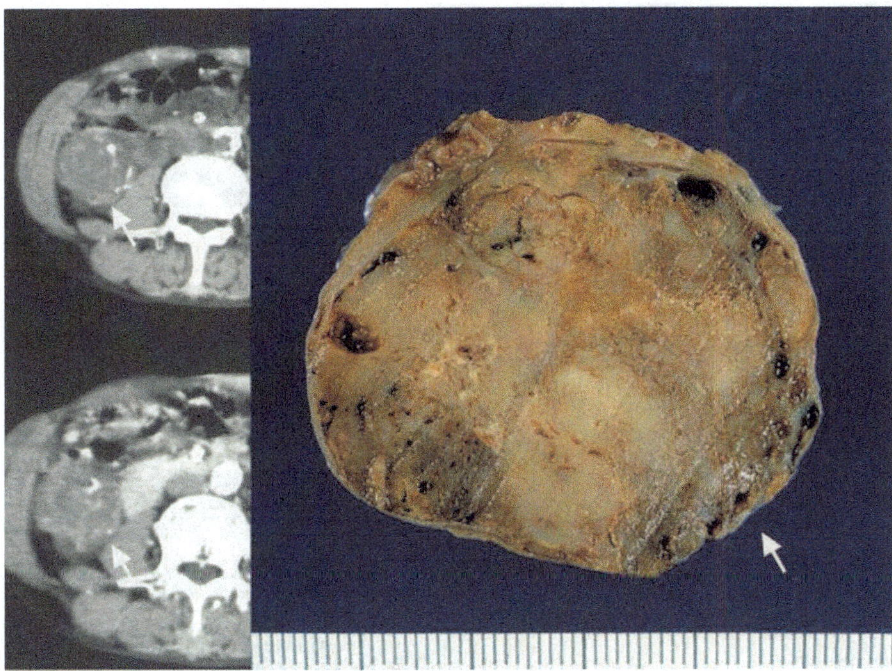

Fig. 123. Case 26. A 64-year-old man who might possibly have chronic glomerulonephritis, and who had a 13-year history of dialysis. This was a case of papillary renal cell carcinoma and multiple cancers. Nephrectomy, thyroidectomy, and parathyroidectomy were performed because of thyroid cancer and secondary hyperparathyroidism. Papillary renal cell carcinoma, pT1b,pNx,pMx,G2,INFα,v(−)

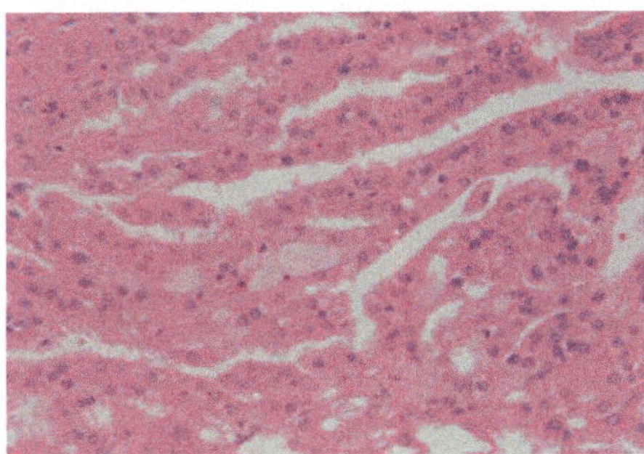

Fig. 124. Case 26. HE stain, ×200

Case 28. A 52-year-old man (the same patient as in Case 10) with chronic glomerulonephritis and with a history of dialysis of 14 years and 6 months. Renal cell carcinomas developed in the left kidney 9 years after right nephrectomy due to renal cell carcinoma (Figs. 127 and 128). A mass about 5 mm in diameter was observed in the cyst wall (indicated by a white arrow in the left upper panel and a white arrow in the upper part of the right panel), and contrast enhancement was noted. The primary

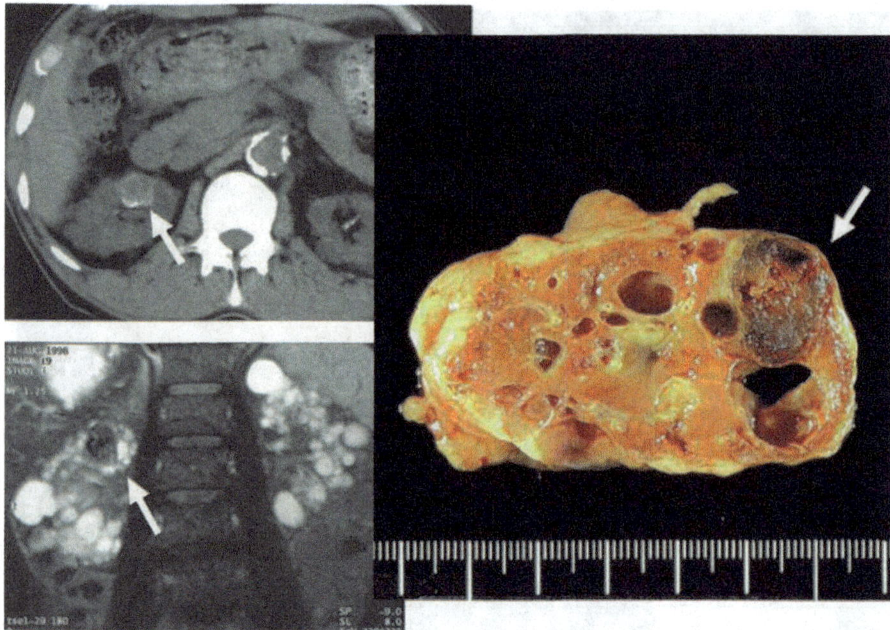

FIG. 125. Case 27. A 68-year-old man with chronic glomerulonephritis and with a history of dialysis of 13 years and 6 months. Renal cell carcinoma was suspected before death, and clear cell carcinoma was found at autopsy. Clear cell carcinoma, pT1a,pN0,pM0,G1,INFα,v(−)

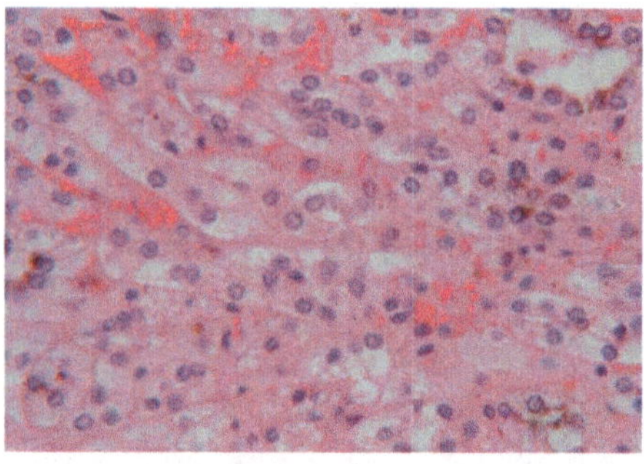

FIG. 126. Case 27. HE stain, ×400

renal cell carcinoma (surrounded by white arrows) was observed in the hilum of the kidney, and part of it protruded into the renal pelvis (blue arrow). Although not diagnosed by imaging techniques, there was another renal cell carcinoma of 8 mm in diameter, and the disease was multiple and bilateral.

Case 29. A 40-year-old man with chronic glomerulonephritis and with a history of dialysis of 15 years and 8 months. In this patient, who had a long history of dialysis, the renal cell carcinoma was surrounded by many cysts, did not protrude from the renal margin, and was hypovascular on dynamic CT, so the diagnosis was difficult (Figs. 129 and 130). The disease was papillary renal cell carcinoma.

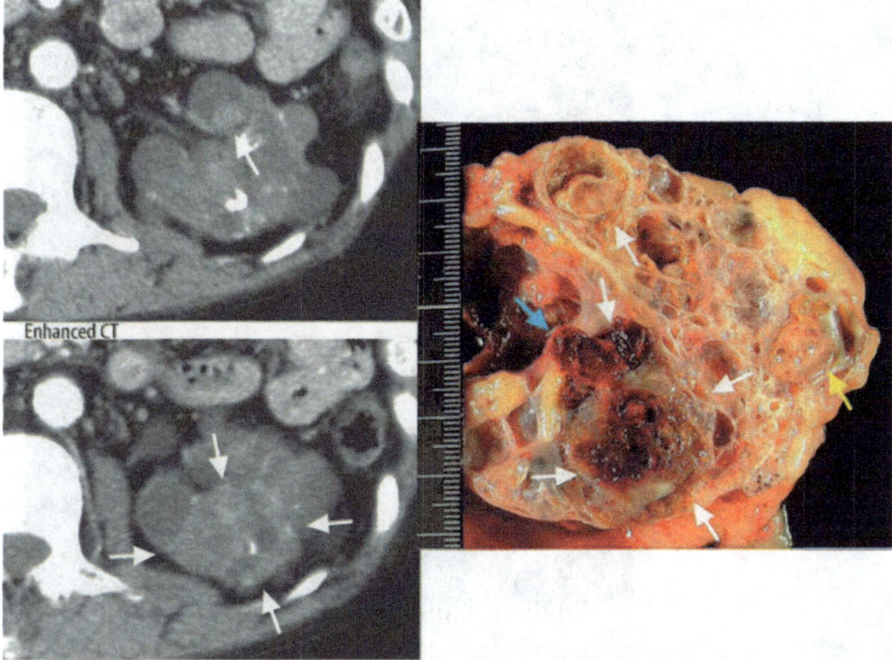

FIG. 127. Case 28. A 52-year-old man (the same patient as Case 10) with chronic glomerulonephritis 9 years after right nephrectomy, and with a history of dialysis of 14 years and 6 months.
Renal cell carcinoma was found in the other kidney 9 years after unilateral nephrectomy for
renal cell carcinoma. The renal cell carcinoma was exposed in the renal pelvis. Papillary renal
cell carcinoma, pT1a,pNx,pMx,G2,INFβ,v(−) (CT in the lower panel: Reproduced from [6], by
permission of Oxford University Press)

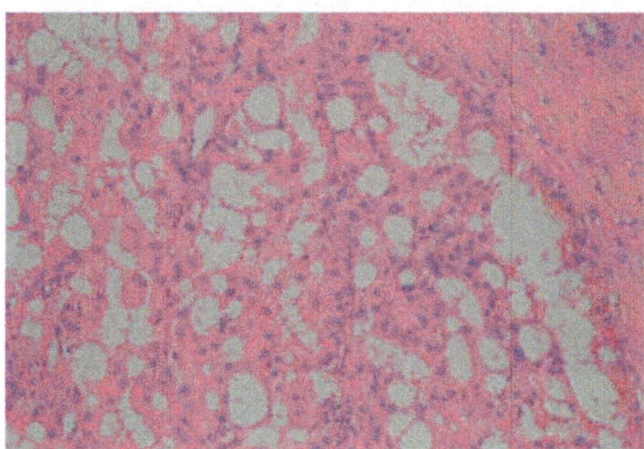

FIG. 128. Case 28. HE stain, ×200

Case 30. A 31-year-old man with chronic glomerulonephritis and with a history of
dialysis of 15 years and 9 months. A papillary renal cell carcinoma 4.5 cm in diameter
appeared in the lower pole of the left kidney after a 9-year follow-up, and nephrectomy was performed. The renal cell carcinoma was surrounded by many cysts, did
not protrude from the renal margin, showed no marked contrast enhancement, and
was hypovascular (Figs. 131 and 132). Simple nephrectomy was performed. Renal

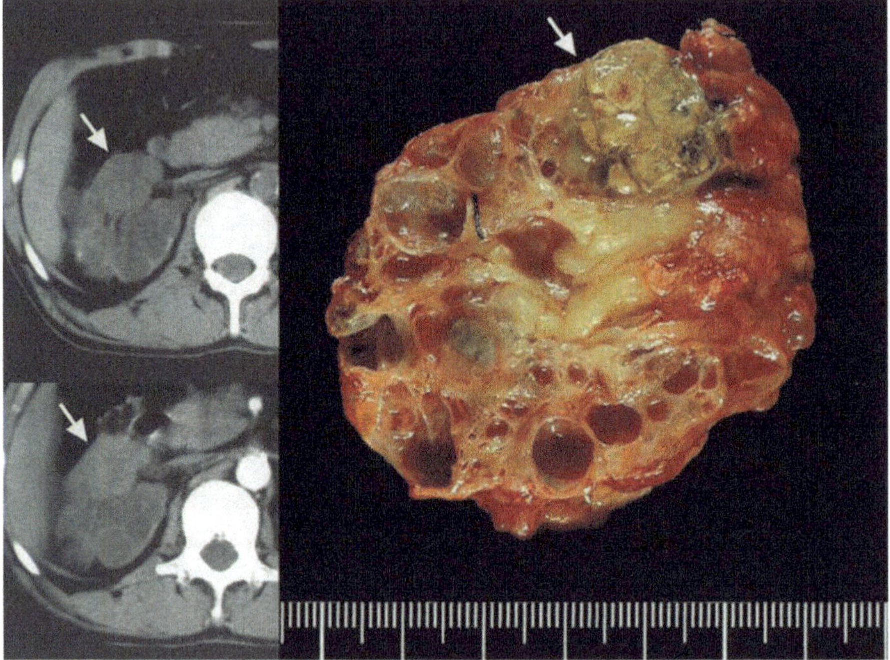

Fig. 129. Case 29. A 40-year-old man with chronic glomerulonephritis and with a history of dialysis of 15 years and 8 months. This was a case of papillary renal cell carcinoma not protruding from the renal margin. Papillary renal cell carcinoma, pT1a,pNx,pMx,G1>>2,INFα,v(−) (CT in the lower panel: Reproduced from [6], by permission of Oxford University Press)

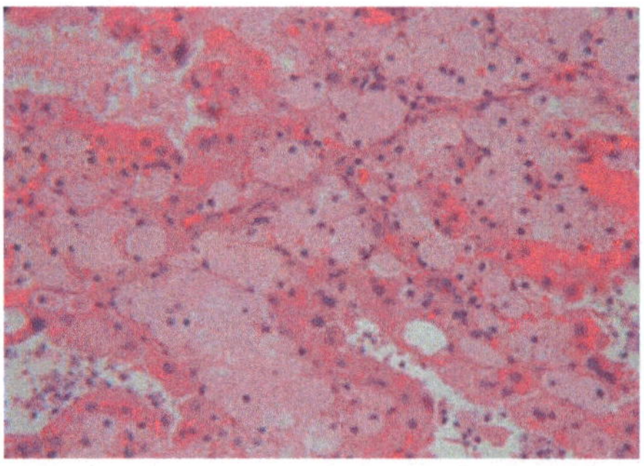

Fig. 130. Case 29. HE stain, ×200

cell carcinoma recurred at the site of the nephrectomy after 9 years and 4 months (Case 34).

Case 31. A 77-year-old man with chronic glomerulonephritis, and with a history of CAPD of 11-years and a history of hemodialysis of 8 years and 10 months. Renal cell carcinoma was suspected while the patient was receiving CAPD and hemodialysis, but he died from encapsulated peritoneal sclerosis. Papillary renal cell carcinoma and nonpapillary renal cell carcinoma were found at autopsy (Figs. 133 and 134). Acquired

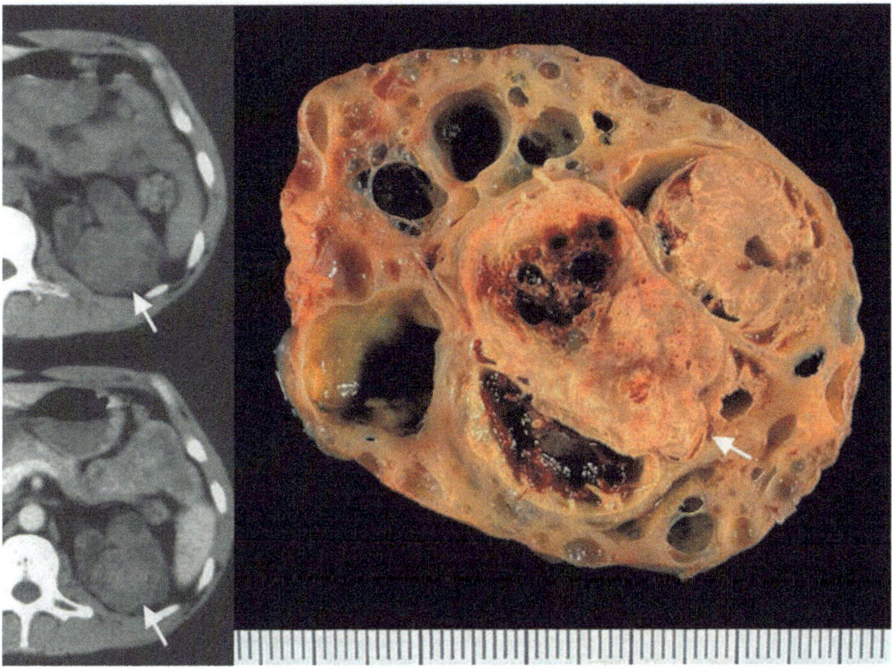

Fig. 131. Case 30. A 31-year-old man with chronic glomerulonephritis and with a history of dialysis of 15 years and 9 months. A renal cell carcinoma 4.5 cm in diameter (not protruding from the renal margin) occurred in the lower pole of the left kidney after a 9-year follow-up. Renal cell carcinoma recurred at the site of resection after 9 years and 4 months (Case 34). Papillary renal cell carcinoma, pT1b,pNx,pMx,G2,INFα,v(−) (Reproduced from [34], with permission from Elsevier Inc.)

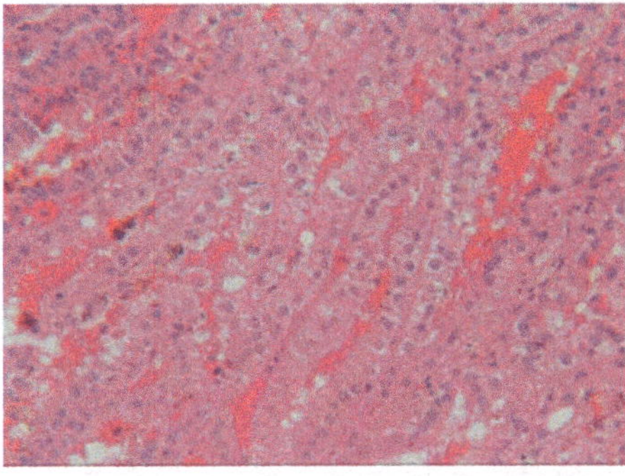

Fig. 132. Case 30. HE stain, ×400

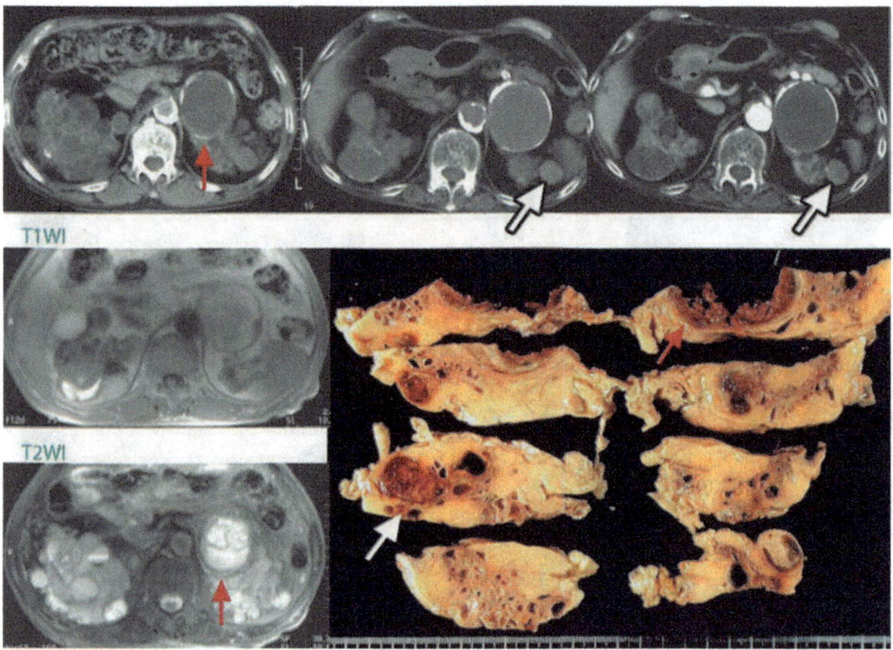

FIG. 133. Case 31. A 77-year-old man with chronic glomerulonephritis, with a history of CAPD of 11 years and a history of hemodialysis of 8 years and 10 months. Renal cell carcinoma was suspected while the patient was receiving CAPD and hemodialysis. Papillary and nonpapillary renal cell carcinomas were found at autopsy after death from encapsulated peritoneal sclerosis. Papillary renal cell carcinoma, pT1a,pN0,pM0,G1,INFα,v(−)

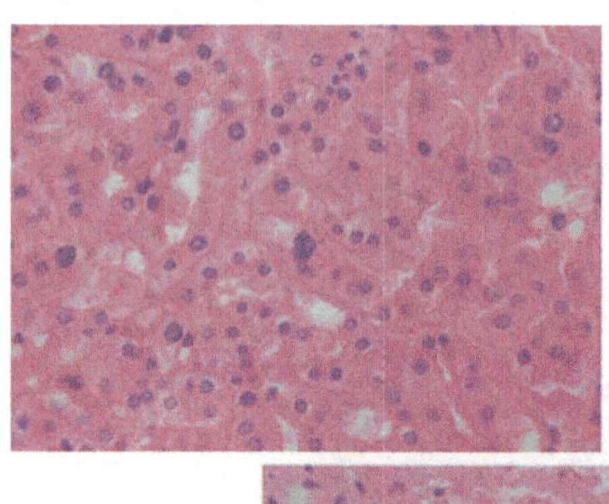

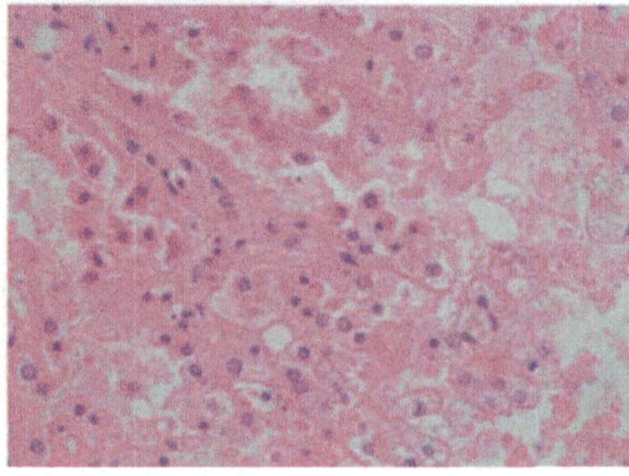

FIG. 134. Case 31. HE stain: *top*, ×400; *bottom*, ×200

cystic disease of the kidney and left renal hematoma (5 cm) strongly suggested renal cell carcinoma, and the patient had been followed up. The primary tumor (papillary renal cell carcinoma) was found in the left kidney (white arrows), a clear cell carcinoma was found in the wall of a very large cyst (red arrows), and a clear cell carcinoma was also found in the right kidney. This case is an example of the extreme difficulty of diagnosing small renal cell carcinoma in kidneys with markedly advanced acquired cystic disease of the kidney.

Case 32. A 59-year-old man with chronic glomerulonephritis and with a history of dialysis of 21 years and 3 months. A renal cell carcinoma had metastasized to the lymph nodes (Figs. 135 and 136). In this patient with a long history of dialysis, a mass in the left kidney (white arrows) and a very large lymph node metastasis (yellow arrows) were found. Both the mass in the left kidney and the very large lymph node metastasis showed little contrast enhancement on dynamic CT and were hypovascular.

Case 33. A 50-year-old man with chronic glomerulonephritis and with a history of dialysis of 21 years and 5 months. Renal cell carcinoma was detected because of the presence of hematuria. Papillary renal cell carcinoma developed in the wall of a very large hematoma in the left kidney, and spindle cell carcinoma occurred simultaneously above the first tumor [50] (Figs. 137 and 138). The patient died from metastasis of a spindle cell carcinoma. A hemorrhagic cyst with a calcified wall 10 cm in diameter

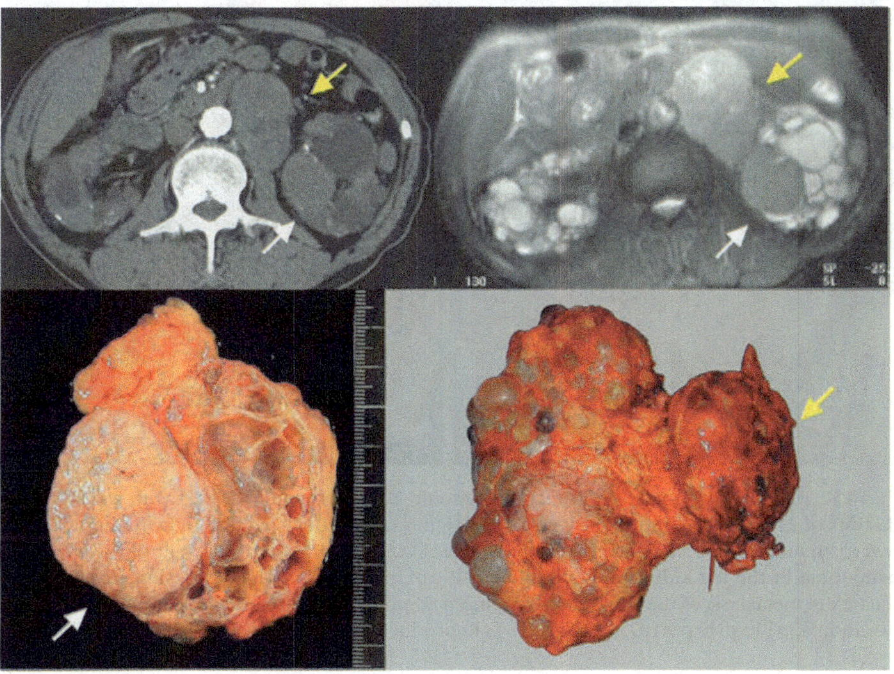

FIG. 135. Case 32. A 59-year-old man with chronic glomerulonephritis and with a history of dialysis of 21 years and 3 months. The renal cell carcinoma metastasized to lymph nodes. Granular cell carcinoma, pT1b,pN1,pM0,G2,INFα,v(−)

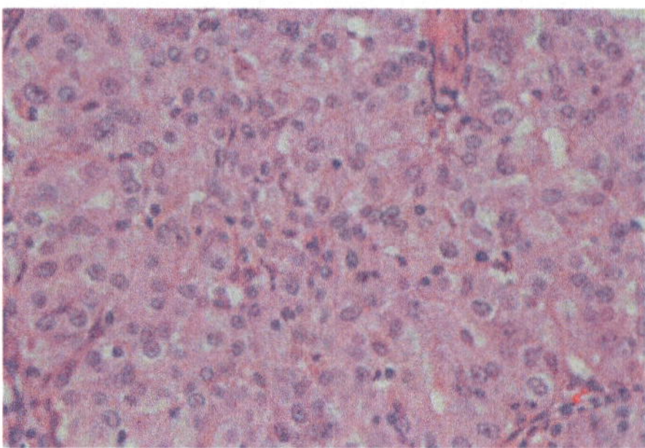

Fig. 136. Case 32. HE stain, ×400

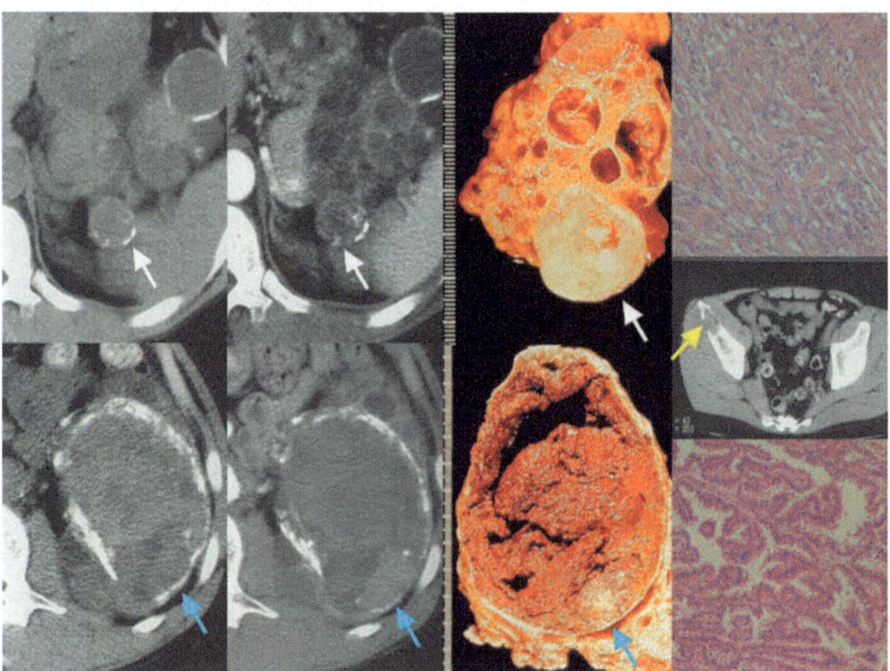

Fig. 137. Case 33. A 50-year-old man with chronic glomerulonephritis and with a history of dialysis of 21 years and 5 months. Renal cell carcinoma was detected due to hematuria. There was a simultaneous occurrence of a papillary renal cell carcinoma in the wall of a very large hematoma in the left kidney and a spindle cell carcinoma above the first lesion. The patient died from metastasis of the spindle cell carcinoma. Spindle cell carcinoma + papillary renal cell carcinoma, pT1a,pN0,pM1,G3>2,INFβ,v(−) (Reproduced from [50], with permission)

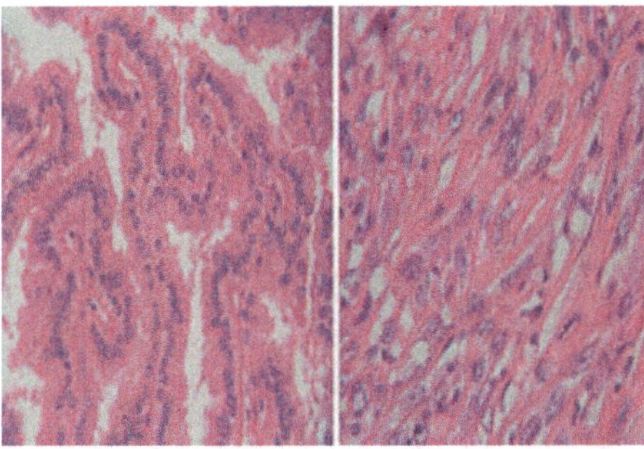

FIG. 138. Case 33. *Right*. Spindle cell carcinoma. HE stain, ×400. *Left*. Papillary renal cell carcinoma. HE stain, ×200

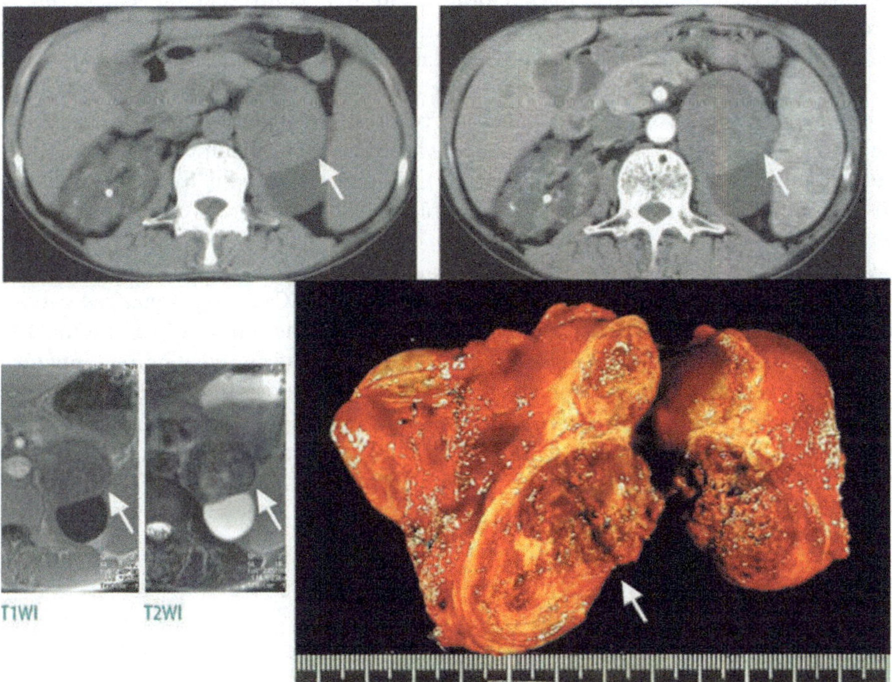

FIG. 139. Case 34. A 41-year-old man with chronic glomerulonephritis and with a history of dialysis of 25 years and 1 month (the same patient as Case 30). This is a possible recurrence at the same site 9 years and 4 months after the resection of renal cell carcinoma. Papillary renal cell carcinoma, pT1b,pNx,pMx,G2,INFα,v(−) (Reproduced from [132], by permission of Oxford University Press)

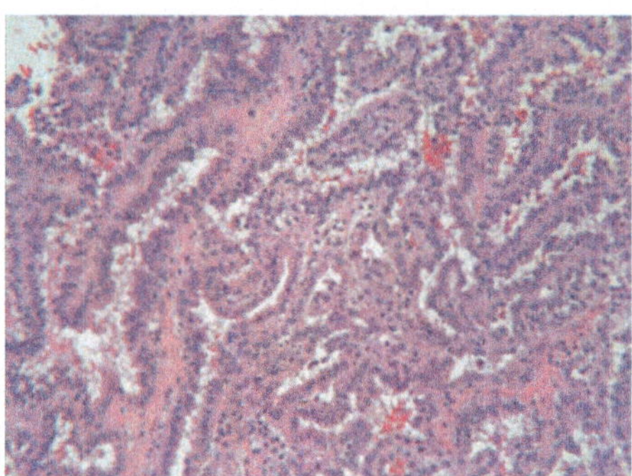

Fig. 140. Case 34. HE stain, ×100

was observed near the hilum of the left kidney, and slight contrast enhancement (blue arrows) was noted on helical dynamic CT. A diagnosis of renal cell carcinoma was made, surgery was performed, and a papillary renal cell carcinoma was disclosed which was similar to that found in the first clinical case in the world. A mass 3.0 cm in diameter (white arrows) that showed no contrast enhancement was observed in the upper pole, and this white tumor (upper white arrow) was spindle cell carcinoma and had metastasized to bone (yellow arrow). This case shows the difficulty of diagnosing spindle cell carcinoma even by contrast-enhanced CT, as well as the importance of screening.

Case 34. A 41-year-old man with chronic glomerulonephritis and with a history of dialysis of 25 years and 1 month (the same patient as Case 30). Renal cell carcinoma appeared to have occurred at the site of a previous renal cell carcinoma 10 years after its resection [132] (Figs. 139 and 140). Following simple nephrectomy for papillary renal cell carcinoma, a mass appeared at the same site and became enlarged, and another operation was required. The mass showed slight contrast enhancement on CT. The tumor was inconspicuous in T1- or T2-weighted MR images, but the signal level of the cysts was low on T1-weighted imaging and high on T2-weighted imaging.

Postscript

This book, *Acquired Cystic Disease of the Kidney and Renal Cell Carcinoma: Complications of Long-Term Dialysis*, is a compilation of the cases that I have encountered to date, including the world's first clinical case, the results of a follow-up which continued for more than two decades, nationwide questionnaire surveys which were carried out during the past 24 years, and the results of our studies on the etiology of the disease. The history of this research is summarized in Table 17.

Figure 141 is a photograph taken at the residence of Prince Takamatsu on the occasion of the 18th International Cancer Symposium subsidized by the Princess Takamatsu Cancer Research Fund (November 17–19, 1987, Tokyo). Princess Takamatsu, Dr. Knudson, who proposed the multistep theory of oncogenesis, and Dr. Li, who described Li-Fraumeni syndrome, are seen in the photograph. Figure 142 is a wooden cup with the family emblem of Prince Takamatsu, which was given in memory of this event.

Figure 143 is a commemorative photograph of the participants in the U.S.–Japan Symposium on Cancer of the Kidney (February 18–19, 1991, East-West Center, Honolulu, Hawaii) surrounding Prince Hitachi.

In addition to the presentations at these international conferences, I have delivered educational lectures at the conferences of the Japanese Society for Dialysis Therapy, and 38 lectures at dialysis symposia throughout Japan.

Acknowledgments. This book would never have been completed without the tireless efforts of many people, including fellow members of my department, doctors from related hospitals, dialysis facilities, and urology departments in various parts of Japan who kindly cooperated in the questionnaires, and investigators who provided the research material. I would like to express my gratitude by acknowledging their contributions here.

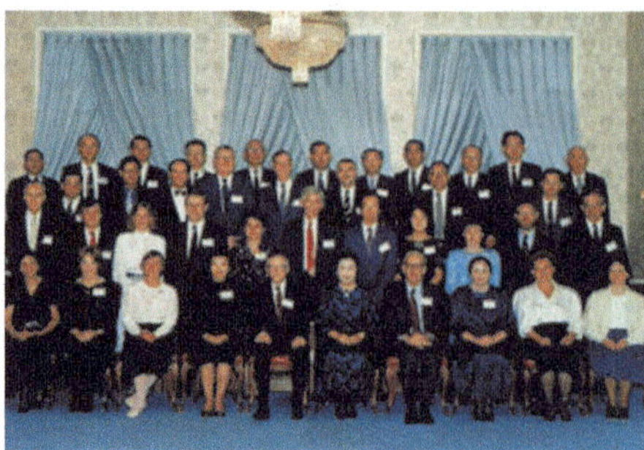

Fig. 141. A commemorative photograph taken at the 18th International Conference on Cancer subsidized by the Princess Takamatsu Cancer Fund (at the residence of Prince Takamatsu)

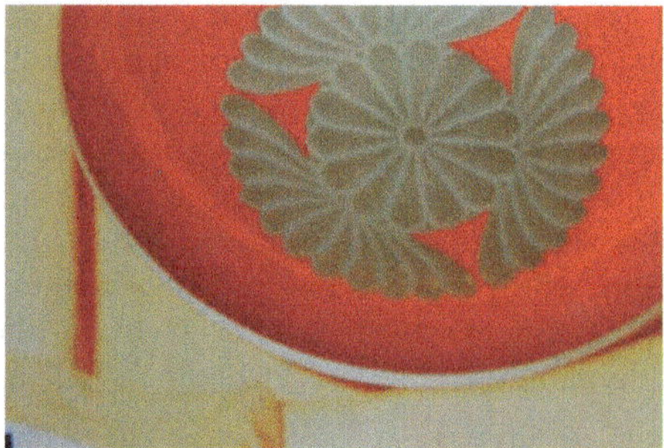

Fig. 142. Wooden cup with the family emblem of Prince Takamatsu, which was presented on this occasion

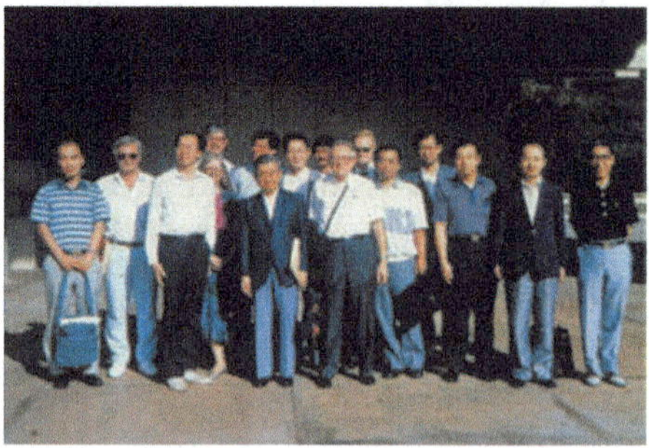

Fig. 143. A commemorative photograph taken at the Japan–U.S. Cancer Symposium in Hawaii, Campus of the University of Hawaii

Brief History of the Author

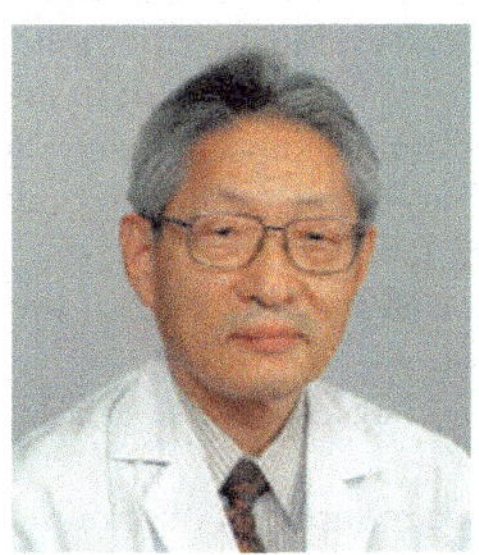

1965: Graduated from the Kanazawa University School of Medicine.

1970: Completed a course in the Department of Medical Research, Kanazawa University Graduate School (First Department of Internal Medicine, instructed by Prof. Takeuchi), and obtained a doctorate of medicine (PhD).

1972–1973: Joined kidney disease study activities as a fellow at Mt. Sinai Hospital of Cleveland in the United States.

1973–1975: Studied under Prof. Hollenberg and Prof. Merrill at Peter Bent Brigham (the present Brigham and Women's) Hospital (Boston) and the School of Medicine, Harvard University, in the United States.

1975: After returning to Japan, took office as an associate professor in the Department of Nephrology, Kanazawa Medical University.

April 1989: Took office as a professor in the Department of Nephrology, Kanazawa Medical University, and as a professor at the Medical Research Institute.

September 1994: Took office as the chief professor in the Department of Nephrology, Kanazawa Medical University.

April 2004: After a departmental reorganization, took office as a professor in the Department of Kidney Function Therapeutics (Nephrology), Kanazawa Medical University.

March 2006: Retired at the normal retirement age.

April 2006: Emeritus professor of Kanazawa Medical University and Division of Nephrology, Asanogawa General Hospital.

TABLE 17. Progress in research into acquired cystic disease of the kidney and renal cell carcinoma

1972 While I studied in the United States, I was taught that "cysts eventually develop in all end-stage kidneys"

1977 Dunnill et al. [1] reported from observation of an autopsy that acquired renal cysts and renal cell carcinoma develop in long-term hemodialysis patients

1978 We experienced the world's first clinical case of acquired renal cysts and renal cell carcinoma, which had developed in a long-term hemodialysis patient (Nippon Jinzo Gakkai Shi (Jpn J Nephrol) 1979, 21: 1145)

1980 We reported that "A diseased kidney becomes smaller 3 years after the start of hemodialysis, and thereafter become larger because of the development of acquired cysts. Sometimes a renal cell carcinoma develops in the acquired cystic disease" [2]

TABLE 17. *Continued*

1982 We started a nation-wide questionnaire study on renal cell carcinoma in dialysis patients [55]

1983 Acquired cysts regress after successful renal transplantation [44]

1984 Acquired cysts develop in continuous ambulatory peritoneal dialysis (CAPD) patients [38]

1985 The development of acquired cysts is more prevalent in male patients [37]

1985–1989 Acquired cysts are derived from proximal tubules [26–29]

1989 When a renal graft fails to function, it causes the development of more acquired cysts in the native kidneys than in the failed graft [54]

1990 A 10-year follow-up study of acquired cystic disease of the kidney in 96 hemodialysis patients with glomerulonephritis [34]

1991 After renal transplantation, acquired cystic disease can develop in the native kidneys in some patients [49]

1991 There is no difference in the rate of development of acquired renal cysts according to the dialysis modality (hemodialysis or CAPD) [41]

1993 The frequency of papillary renal cell carcinoma is high in hemodialysis patients with renal cell carcinoma [62]

1993 A karyotypic study on a hemodialysis patient with papillary renal cell carcinoma [118]

1996 A cytogenetic study of renal cell carcinoma in hemodialysis patients [117]

1997 A 15-year follow-up for acquired cystic disease of the kidney in 96 hemodialysis patients with glomerulonephritis [40]

1998 The recurrence of renal cell carcinoma in a resected hemodialysis patient [132]

2000 Acquired renal cysts communicate more frequently with renal tubules than do renal cysts in autosomal dominant polycystic kidney disease (ADPKD) [30]

2000 From a study of renal biopsies, it was found that acquired renal cysts start to develop after only a mild reduction of renal function [25]

2003 A 20-year follow-up study of acquired cystic disease of the kidney in 96 hemodialysis patients with glomerulonephritis [13]

2004 The outcome for renal cell carcinoma is better when it is detected by screening than by symptoms [105]

2005 The results of a questionnaire study in 2004 and a review of past questionnaires is published [63]

References

1. Dunnill MS, Millard PR, Oliver D (1977) Acquired cystic disease of the kidneys: a hazard of long-term intermittent maintenance haemodialysis. J Clin Pathol 30:868–877
2. Ishikawa I, Saito Y, Onouchi Z, Kitada H, Suzuki S, Kurihara S, Yuri T, Shinoda A (1980) Development of acquired cystic disease and adenocarcinoma of the kidney in glomerulonephritic chronic hemodialysis patients. Clin Nephrol 14:1–6
3. Grantham JJ (1990) Polycystic kidney disease: neoplasia in disguise. Am J Kidney Dis 15:110–116
4. Ishikawa I (1990) Acquired renal cystic disease. In: Gardner KD Jr, Bernstein J (eds) The cystic kidney. Kluwer Academic, London, pp 351–377
5. Ishikawa I (1999) Acquired cystic disease and renal tumors in long-term dialysis patients. In: Brown E, Parfrey P (eds) Complications of long-term dialysis. Oxford University Press, Oxford, pp 145–169
6. Ishikawa I (2005) Cancer in dialysis patients. In: Cohen EP (ed) Cancer and the kidney. Oxford University Press, Oxford, pp 227–247
7. Ishikawa I (1988) Development of adenocarcinoma and acquired cystic disease of the kidney in hemodialysis patients. In: Miller RW, Watanabe S, Fraumeri JF Jr, Sugimura T, Takayama S, Sugano H (eds) Unusual occurrences as clues to cancer etiology. Japan Scientific Societies Press, Tokyo, pp 77–86
8. Ishikawa I (1999) Renal cell carcinomas in patients on long-term hemodialysis. Contrib Nephrol 128:28–44
9. Ishikawa I (1984) Acquired renal cystic disease (Ta-nouhouka-isyukujin). Jin-To-Tohseki (Kidney Dial) 17:341–348
10. Ishikawa I (1991) Acquired cystic disease: mechanisms and manifestations. Semin Nephrol 11:671–684
11. Ishikawa I (1991) Uremic acquired renal cystic disease. Natural history and complications. Nephron 58:257–267
12. Kyushu Pediatric Nephrology Study Group (1999) Acquired cystic kidney disease in children undergoing continuous ambulatory peritoneal dialysis. Am J Kidney Dis 34:242–246
13. Ishikawa I, Saito Y, Asaka M, Tomosugi N, Yuri T, Watanabe M, Honda R (2003) Twenty-year follow-up of acquired renal cystic disease. Clin Nephrol 59:153–159
14. Ishikawa I (1985) Uremic acquired cystic disease of kidney. Urology 26:101–108
15. Jabour BA, Ralls PW, Tang WW, Boswell WDJ, Colletti PM, Feinstein EI, Massry SG (1987) Acquired cystic disease of the kidneys. Computed tomography and ultrasonography appraisal in patients on peritoneal and hemodialysis. Invest Radiol 22:728–732

16. Levine E, Grantham JJ, Slusher SL, Greathouse JL, Krohn BP (1984) CT of acquired cystic kidney disease and renal tumors in long-term dialysis patients. AJR 142:125–131
17. Mickisch O, Bommer J, Bachmann S, Waldherr R, Mann JFE, Ritz E (1984) Multicystic transformation of kidneys in chronic renal failure. Nephron 38:93–99
18. Smith JW, Sallman AL, Williamson MR, Lott CG (1987) Acquired renal cystic disease: two cases of associated adenocarcinoma and a renal ultrasound survey of a peritoneal dialysis population. Am J Kidney Dis 10:41–46
19. Ishikawa I, Shikura N, Horiguchi T, Morimoto S, Tamai Y, Masuzaki S, Shinoda A (1988) Size distribution of acquired cysts in chronic hemodialysis patients. J Kanazawa Med Univ 13:171–175
20. Gehrig JJJ, Gottheiner TI, Swenson RS (1985) Acquired cystic disease of the end-stage kidney. Am J Med 79:609–620
21. Feiner HD, Katz LA, Gallo GR (1981) Acquired cystic disease of kidney in chronic dialysis patients. Urology 17:260–264
22. Watanabe M, Ishikawa I (2005) Kidney volume and development of acquired cystic disease of the kidney in diabetic nephropathy after the start of hemodialysis (in Japanese with English abstract). J Kanazawa Med Univ 30:191–197
23. Neureiter D, Frank H, Kunzendorf U, Waldherr R, Amann K (2002) Dialysis-associated acquired cystic kidney disease imitating autosomal dominant polycystic kidney disease in a patient receiving long-term peritoneal dialysis. Nephrol Dial Transplant 17:500–503
24. Ishikawa I (1990) Comparison of cyst characteristics in acquired and inherited renal cystic disease. In: Carone FA, Dobbie JW (eds) Advances in the pathogenesis of polycystic kidney disease. Baxter Healthcare Corporation, Chicago, pp 85–90
25. Liu JS, Ishikawa I, Horiguchi T (2000) Incidence of acquired renal cysts in biopsy specimens. Nephron 84:142–147
26. Ishikawa I (1985) Unusual composition of cyst fluid in acquired cystic disease of the end-stage kidney. Nephron 41:373–374
27. Ishikawa I (1986) Beta-2-microglobulin level of cyst fluid in uremic acquired cystic disease of the kidney. Nephron 44:381
28. Ishikawa I, Horiguchi T, Shikura N (1989) Lectin peroxidase conjugate reactivity in acquired cystic disease of the kidney. Nephron 51:211–214
29. Ishikawa I, Saito Y, Shikura N, Yuri T, Shinoda A, Shiraiwa K, Tsugawa R (1989) Excretion of hippuran into acquired renal cysts in chronic hemodialysis patient. Nephron 52:110–111
30. Liu JS, Ishikawa I (2000) Communication between acquired renal cysts and renal tubules. Nephron 86:243–244
31. Sato A, Uda H, Hata H, Shimizu N, Ohata K (1989) An autopsy case of interlobar arterial dissection of the kidney following long-term hemodialysis. Acta Pathol Jpn 39:342–348
32. Soffer O, Miller LR, Lichtman JB (1987) CT findings in complications of acquired renal cystic disease. J Comput Assist Tomogr 11:905–908
33. Tuttle RJ, Minielly JA, Fay WP (1971) Spontaneous renal hemorrhage in chronic glomerular nephritis and dialysis. Radiology 98:137–138
34. Ishikawa I, Saito Y, Shikura N, Kitada H, Shinoda A, Suzuki S (1990) Ten-year prospective study on the development of renal cell carcinoma in dialysis patients. Am J Kidney Dis 16:452–458
35. Ishikawa I, Saito Y, Kitada H, Onouchi Z, Shinoda A (1980) Computed tomography of kidneys with hemodialysis. J Kanazawa Med Univ 5:146–154
36. Ishikawa I, Saito Y, Fukuda Y, Ishii H, Asaka M, Tomosugi N, Yuri T (1997) Relationship between cyst enlargement in acquired renal cystic disease and erythropoietin concentration or hematocrit level (Japanese abstract). Nippon Jinzo Gakkai Shi (Jpn J Nephrol) 39:227

37. Ishikawa I, Onouchi Z, Saito Y, Tateishi K, Shinoda A, Suzuki S, Kitada H, Sugishita N, Fukuda Y (1985) Sex differences in acquired cystic disease of the kidney on long-term dialysis. Nephron 39:336–340

38. Ishikawa I, Moncrief JW, Aguirre F, Brindley BW, Mott CL (1984) Acquired cystic kidney disease in continuous ambulatory peritoneal dialysis patients. In: Maekawa M, Norph KD, Kishimoto T, Moncrief JW (eds) Machine-free dialysis for patient convenience. ISAO Press, Cleveland, pp 131–133

39. Ishikawa I (1992) Acquired renal cystic disease and its complications in continuous ambulatory peritoneal dialysis patients. Perit Dial Int 12:292–297

40. Ishikawa I, Saito Y, Nakamura M, Takada K, Ishii H, Nakazawa T, Fukuda Y, Asaka M, Tomosugi N, Yuri T (1997) Fifteen-year follow-up of acquired renal cystic disease: a gender difference. Nephron 75:315–320

41. Ishikawa I, Shikura N, Nagahara M, Shinoda A, Saito Y (1991) Comparison of severity of acquired renal cysts between CAPD and hemodialysis. Adv Perit Dial 7: 91–95

42. Ishikawa I, Fukuda Y, Takada K, Ishii H, Nakamura M, Asaka M, Tomosugi N, Yuri T (1996) Is progression of acquired cystic disease affected by the dialyzer membrane (Japanese abstract)? J Jpn Soc Dial Ther 29(S1):709

43. Ishikawa I, Yamaya H, Nakamura M, Sakamoto S, Asaka M, Tomosugi N, Yuri T (1996) Erythropoietin does not affect the development and progression of acquired renal cystic disease. Nephrol Dial Transplant 11:A262

44. Ishikawa I, Yuri T, Kitada H, Shinoda A (1983) Regression of acquired cystic disease of the kidney after successful renal transplantation. Am J Nephrol 3:310–314

45. Morita K, Ishikawa I, Hayama S, Adachi H, Sato K, Nakagawa T, Yamaya H, Asaka M, Tomosugi N, Yuri T (2004) Early regression of acquired renal cysts after renal transplantation. Presented at the Tohkai–Hokuriku Renal Failure Conference (Nagoya), March 20, 2004

46. Klotz LH, Kulkarni C, Mills G (1991) End stage renal disease serum contains a specific renal cell growth factor. J Urol 145:156–160

47. Lien YH, Hunt KR, Siskind MS, Zukoski C (1993) Association of cyclosporin A with acquired cystic kidney disease of the native kidneys in renal transplant recipients. Kidney Int 44:613–616

48. Ishikawa I, Nakazawa T, Asaka M, Yuri T, Tomosugi N (1998) Cyclosporine effect on volume of original kidney and acquired cysts after renal transplantation (Japanese abstract). Nippon Jinzo Gakkai Shi (Jpn J Nephrol) 40:189

49. Ishikawa I, Shikura N, Shinoda A (1991) Cystic transformation in native kidneys in renal allograft recipients with long-standing good function. Am J Nephrol 11:217–223

50. Ishikawa I, Yamaya H (2002) Sarcomatoid renal cell carcinoma in dialysis patients (in Japanese). Jpn J Clin Dial (Tokyo) 18:347–353

51. Hayama S, Ishikawa I, Yamaya H, Asaka M, Tomosugi N, Yuri T, Miyazawa K, Suzuki K, Ueda Y (2004) Renal cell carcinoma in original kidney detected by periodic screening for malignancy after renal transplantation (young female case) (Japanese abstract). Nippon Jinzo Gakkai Shi (Jpn J Nephrol) 46:515

52. Ishikawa I, Ishii H, Shinoda A, Tateishi K, Ben A, Suzuki K, Tsugawa R (1991) Renal cell carcinoma of the native kidney after renal transplantation. A case report and review of the literature. Nephron 58:354–358

53. Ishikawa I (1992) Acquired cysts and neoplasms of the kidneys in renal allograft recipients. Contrib Nephrol 100:254–268

54. Ishikawa I, Shikura N, Kitada H, Yuri T, Shinoda A, Nakazawa T (1989) Severity of acquired renal cysts in native kidneys and renal allograft with long-standing poor function. Am J Kidney Dis 14:18–24

55. Ishikawa I, Shinoda A (1983) Renal adenocarcinoma with or without acquired cysts in chronic hemodialysis patients. Clin Nephrol 20:321–322

56. Denton MD, Magee CC, Ovuworie C, Mauiyyedi S, Pascual M, Colvin RB, Cosimi AB, Tolkoff-Rubin N (2002) Prevalence of renal cell carcinoma in patients with ESRD pre-transplantation: a pathologic analysis. Kidney Int 61:2201–2209

57. Ishikawa I (1991) Renal cell carcinoma in chronic hemodialysis patients: a 1990 questionnaire study and review of past questionnaires (in Japanese with English abstract). J Jpn Soc Dial Ther 24:493–497

58. Ishikawa I (2002) Prognosis in dialysis patients complicated with renal cell carcinoma (in Japanese with English abstract). J Jpn Soc Dial Ther 35:287–293

59. Horiguchi T, Ishikawa I (1993) Immunohistochemical study in acquired cystic disease of the kidney: expression of vimentin, epidermal growth factor, epidermal growth factor receptor and c-erb B2 gene product (in Japanese with English abstract). Nippon Jinzo Gakkai Shi (Jpn J Nephrol) 35:797–807

60. Herrera GA (1991) C-erb B-2 amplification in cystic renal disease. Kidney Int 40:509–513

61. Takebayashi S, Hidai H, Chiba T, Irisawa M, Matsubara S (2000) Renal cell carcinoma in acquired cystic kidney disease: volume growth rate determined by helical computed tomography. Am J Kidney Dis 36:759–766

62. Ishikawa I, Kovacs G (1993) High incidence of papillary renal cell tumours in patients on chronic haemodialysis. Histopathology 22:135–139

63. Ishikawa I (2005) Present status of renal cell carcinoma in dialysis patients: a questionnaire study in 2004 and review of past questionnaires since 1982 (in Japanese with English abstract). J Jpn Soc Dial Ther 38:1689–1700

64. Lu TC, Lim PS, Hsu WM, Wang TH, Liu ST (2001) Renal oncocytoma in acquired renal cystic disease. J Formos Med Assoc 100:488–491

65. Makita Y, Inenaga T, Kinjo M, Komatsu K, Onoyama K, Fujishima M (1991) Renal oncocytoma developed in a long-term hemodialysis patient. Nephron 57:355–357

66. Hanada T, Mimata H, Ohno H, Nasu N, Nakagawa M, Nomura Y (1998) Erythropoietin-producing renal cell carcinoma arising from acquired cystic disease of the kidney. Int J Urol 5:493–494

67. Suvarna SK, Ahuja M, Brown CB (1994) Sarcomatoid renal cell carcinoma arising in hemodialysis-associated acquired cystic kidney disease presenting with disseminated bone marrow infiltration. Am J Kidney Dis 24:581–585

68. Aita K, Tanimoto A, Fujimoto Y, Momomura S, Takemoto F, Hara S, Matsushita H (2003) Sarcomatoid-collecting duct carcinoma arising in hemodialysis-associated acquired cystic kidney: an autopsy report. Pathol Int 53:463–467

69. Fujimori A, Naito H, Miyazaki T, Azuma M, Hashimoto S, Horikawa S (1995) Autopsy findings of a long-term (25 years) hemodialysis case with sarcomatoid renal cell carcinoma (in Japanese with English abstract). J Jpn Soc Dial Ther 28:1273–1277

70. Fujita K, Kajiwara T, Yamada D, Endo M, Furuya T, Kaneko S, Horibe Y, Ishii Y (2003) Sarcomatoid renal cell carcinoma arising in hemodialysis-associated acquired cystic disease of the kidney (in Japanese with English abstract). J Jpn Soc Dial Ther 36:1289–1293

71. Kamoshida T, Yamada S, Saito K, Miura K, Ando Y, Takada S, Honma S, Tabei K, Kusano E, Asano Y (1993) Two autopsy cases of sarcomatoid renal cell carcinoma arising in acquired cystic disease of the kidney, accompanied with M-proteinemia (in Japanese with English abstract). Pathol Clin (Tokyo) 11:739–744

72. Ishikawa I, Saito A, Chikazawa Y, Asaka M, Tomosugi N, Yuri T, Suzuki K, Ueda Y, Ozaki M (2003) Cystic renal cell carcinoma, suspected because of lack of regression of renal cysts after renal transplantation in a dialysis patient with acquired renal cystic disease. Clin Exp Nephrol 7:81–84

73. Chung-Park M, Ricanati E, Lankerani M, Kedia K (1983) Acquired renal cysts and multiple renal cell and urothelial tumors. Am J Clin Pathol 79:238–242

74. Satoh S, Tsuchiya N, Habuchi T, Ishiyama T, Seimo K, Kato T (2005) Renal cell and transitional cell carcinoma in a Japanese population undergoing maintenance dialysis. J Urol 174:1749–1753

75. Hughson MD, Hennigar GR, McManus JFA (1980) Atypical cysts, acquired renal cystic disease, and renal cell tumors in end stage dialysis kidneys. Lab Invest 42:475–480

76. Grantham JJ, Levine E (1985) Acquired cystic disease: replacing one kidney disease with another. Kidney Int 28:99–105

77. Segerer S, Meister P (1998) Acquired cystic kidney disease in patients on long-term dialysis: a retrospective study of 125 autopsies. Part 2. Tumors. Pathologe 19:368–372

78. Ishikawa I (1986) Adenocarcinoma of the kidney in chronic hemodialysis patients in Japan. Nationwide questionnaire study and review of case reports. Nippon Jinzo Gakkai Shi (Jpn J Nephrol) 28:1299–1303

79. Ishikawa I (1988) Adenocarcinoma of the kidney in chronic hemodialysis patients in Japan. A 1986 questionnaire study (in Japanese with English abstract). J Jpn Soc Dial Ther 21:465–470

80. Ishikawa I (1989) Renal cell carcinoma in chronic hemodialysis patients in Japan. A 1988 questionnaire study (in Japanese with English abstract). J Jpn Soc Dial Ther 22:639–643

81. Ishikawa I (1993) Renal cell carcinoma in chronic hemodialysis patients. A 1992 questionnaire study (in Japanese with English abstract). J Jpn Soc Dial Ther 26:1355–1362

82. Ishikawa I (1996) Renal cell carcinoma in chronic hemodialysis patients. A 1994 questionnaire study (in Japanese with English abstract). J Jpn Soc Dial Ther 29:109–116

83. Ishikawa I (1998) Renal cell carcinoma in chronic hemodialysis patients. A 1996 questionnaire study (in Japanese with English abstract). J Jpn Soc Dial Ther 31:209–217

84. Ishikawa I (2000) Renal cell carcinoma in chronic hemodialysis patients. A 1998 questionnaire study (in Japanese with English abstract). J Jpn Soc Dial Ther 33:181–188

85. Ishikawa I (2002) Renal cell carcinoma in chronic hemodialysis patients. A questionnaire study in 2000 (in Japanese with English abstract). J Jpn Soc Dial Ther 35:1111–1118

86. Ishikawa I (2004) Present status of renal cell carcinoma in dialysis patients: Questionnaire-based survey in 2002 (in Japanese with English abstract). J Jpn Soc Dial Ther 37:1605–1615

87. Stewart JH, Buccianti G, Agodoa L, Gellert R, McCredie MR, Lowenfels AB, Disney AP, Wolfe RA, Boyle P, Maisonneuve P (2003) Cancers of the kidney and urinary tract in patients on dialysis for end-stage renal disease: analysis of data from the United States, Europe, and Australia and New Zealand. J Am Soc Nephrol 14:197–207

88. Ishikawa I (1988) Adenocarcinoma of the kidney in chronic hemodialysis patients. Int J Artif Organs 11:61–62

89. Ishikawa I (1993) Renal cell carcinoma in chronic hemodialysis patients. A 1990 questionnaire study in Japan. Kidney Int 41:S167–S169

90. Ishikawa I (2004) Present status of renal cell carcinoma in dialysis patients in Japan. Questionnaire study in 2002. Nephron Clin Pract 97:c11–16

91. Maisonneuve P, Agodoa L, Gellert R, Stewart JH, Buccianti G, Lowenfels AB, Wolfe RA, Jones E, Disney AP, Briggs D, McCredie M, Boyle P (1999) Cancer in patients on dialysis for end-stage renal disease: an international collaborative study. Lancet 354:93–99

92. Shikura N, Ishikawa I, Ishii H, Sugishita N, Tateishi K, Shinoda A, Saito Y (1991) Double cancer in dialysis patients (Japanese abstract). J Jpn Soc Dial Ther 24:678

93. Levine E (1992) Renal cell carcinoma in uremic acquired renal cystic disease: incidence, detection, and management. Urol Radiol 13:203–210

94. Ishikawa I (2000) Hemorrhage versus cancer in acquired cystic disease. Semin Dial 13:56

95. Terasawa Y, Suzuki Y, Morita M, Kato M, Suzuki K, Sekino H (1994) Ultrasonic diagnosis of renal cell carcinoma in hemodialysis patients. J Urol 152:846–851

96. Levine E (1995) Renal cell carcinoma: clinical aspects, imaging diagnosis, and staging. Semin Roentgenol 30:128–148

97. Ishikawa I (1982) CT diagnosis in renal diseases (in Japanese). Nankodo, Tokyo, pp 1–206

98. Ishikawa I (2003) How to diagnose RCC surrounded by multiple acquired renal cysts in log-term hemodialysis patient? In: Asano Y (ed) Tips in dialysis therapy (in Japanese). Nakayama Shoten, Tokyo, pp 178–179

99. Takebayashi S, Hidai H, Chiba T, Takagi H, Koike S, Matsubara S (1999) Using helical CT to evaluate renal cell carcinoma in patients undergoing hemodialysis: value of early enhanced images. AJR 172:429–433

100. Suzuki K, Morizono Y, Arai H, Suzuki T, Kubo K, Kanazawa K, Miura A, Matuzaki R, Ozawa S, Maeda H, Koshino K, Nakazawa H, Touma H, Hotta S, Yamaguchi Y (2003) MRI findings of renal cell carcinoma in dialysis patients (correlated with pathology) (in Japanese). J Jpn Assoc Dial Physicians 18:47–60

101. Chandhoke PS, Torrence RJ, Clayman RV, Rothstein M (1992) Acquired cystic disease of the kidney: a management dilemma. J Urol 147:969–974

102. Ishikawa I (1993) Re: acquired cystic disease of the kidney: a management dilemma. J Urol 149:1146–1148

103. Sarasin FP, Wong JB, Levey AS, Meyer KB (1995) Screening for acquired cystic kidney disease: a decision analytic perspective. Kidney Int 48:207–219

104. Choyke PL (2000) Acquired cystic kidney disease. Eur Radiol 10:1716–1721

105. Ishikawa I, Honda R, Yamada Y, Kakuma T (2004) Renal cell carcinoma detected by screening shows better patient survival than that detected following symptoms in dialysis patients. Ther Apher Dial 8:468–473

106. Brown EA (2004) Renal tumours in dialysis patients: who should we screen? Nephron Clin Pract 97:c3–4

107. Isobe Y, Matuura H, Uehira O, Kimura K, Kondo K, Yamada N, Kato N, Ono Y (2004) Two RCCs in original kidney resected by laparoscopic procedure in renal transplantation patients (Japanese abstract). Isyoku (Jpn J Transplant) 39:298–299

108. Takahashi H, Sato M, Kurokawa Y, Sekino S, Fujikura Y, Murayama F, Sekino H (2003) Laparoscopic simple nephrectomy indication and method. Jpn J Clin Dial (Tokyo) 19:811–817

109. Takahashi H, Nozuki M, Usui K, Murayama F, Yumita S, Kurokawa Y, Sekino H (1997) Laparoscopic nephrectomy in two hemodialysis patients with renal cancer (in Japanese). Jin-To-Tohseki (Kidney Dial) 42:259–262

110. Matson MA, Cohen EP (1990) Acquired cystic kidney disease: occurrence, prevalence, and renal cancers. Medicine (Baltimore) 69:217–226

111. Hughson MD, Buchwald D, Fox M (1986) Renal neoplasia and acquired cystic kidney disease in patients receiving long-term dialysis. Arch Pathol Lab Med 110:592–601

112. Miller LR, Soffer O, Nassar VH, Kutner MH (1989) Acquired renal cystic disease in end-stage renal disease: an autopsy study of 155 cases. Am J Nephrol 9:322–328

113. Cheuk W, Lo ES, Chan AK, Chan JK (2002) Atypical epithelial proliferations in acquired renal cystic disease harbor cytogenetic aberrations. Hum Pathol 33:761–765

114. Chudek J, Herbers J, Wilhelm M, Kenck C, Bugert P, Ritz E, Waldman F, Kovacs G (1998) The genetics of renal tumors in end-stage renal failure differs from those occurring in the general population. J Am Soc Nephrol 9:1045–1051

115. Gronwald J, Baur AS, Holtgreve-Grez H, Jauch A, Mosimann F, Jichlinski P, Wauters JP, Cremer T, Guillou L (1999) Chromosomal abnormalities in renal cell neoplasms

associated with acquired renal cystic disease. A series studied by comparative genomic hybridization and fluorescence in situ hybridization. J Pathol 187:308–312

116. Hughson MD, Meloni AM, Silva FG, Sandberg AA (1996) Renal cell carcinoma in an end-stage kidney of a patient with a functional transplant: cytogenetic and molecular genetic findings. Cancer Genet Cytogenet 89:65–68

117. Ishikawa I, Ozaki M, Tominaga Y, Nakamura Y (1996) Cytogenetic abnormalities in renal cell carcinomas associated with uremic acquired renal cystic disease. J Kanazawa Med Univ 21:76–81

118. Ishikawa I, Shikura N, Ozaki M (1993) Papillary renal cell carcinoma with numeric changes of chromosomes in a long-term hemodialysis patient: a karyotype analysis. Am J Kidney Dis 21:553–556

119. Matumoto M, Sakamoto K, Kamura K, Hamano S, Hachisu T, Kenmochi T, Yamada H, Maeda H, Kashiwabara H, Hamaguchi K, Yamada K, Yokoyama T (1995) A case of renal cell carcinoma of the left native kidney following renal transplantation (in Japanese). Isyoku (Jpn J Transplant) 30:605–610

120. Yoshida MA, Shishikura A, Oshima H, Ikeuchi T (1993) Cytogenetic analyses of renal cell carcinoma cells from a patient with chronic renal failure, acquired cystic disease of the kidney and a constitutional chromosome translocation (Japanese abstract). Proceedings of the Japan Cancer Association, 52nd Annual Meeting, p 208

121. Yoshida M, Yao M, Ishikawa I, Kishida T, Nagashima Y, Kondo K, Nakaigawa N, Hosaka M (2002) Somatic von Hippel-Lindau disease gene mutation in clear-cell renal carcinomas associated with end-stage renal disease/acquired cystic disease of the kidney. Genes Chromosomes Cancer 35:359–364

122. Hoshida Y, Nakanishi H, Shin M, Satoh T, Hanai J, Aozasa K (1999) Renal neoplasias in patients receiving dialysis and renal transplantation: clinico-pathological features and p53 gene mutations. Transplantation 68:385–390

123. Yano T, Ito F, Kobayashi K, Yonezawa Y, Suzuki K, Asano R, Hagiwara K, Nakazawa H, Toma H, Yamasaki H (2004) Hypermethylation of the CpG island of connexin 32, a candidate tumor suppressor gene in renal cell carcinomas from hemodialysis patients. Cancer Lett 208:137–142

124. Konda R, Sato H, Hatafuku F, Nozawa T, Ioritani N, Fujioka T (2004) Expression of hepatocyte growth factor and its receptor C-met in acquired renal cystic disease associated with renal cell carcinoma. J Urol 171:2166–2170

125. Ito F, Nakazawa H, Ryoji O, Okuda H, Toma H (2000) Cytokines accumulated in acquired renal cysts in long-term hemodialysis patients. Urol Int 65:21–27

126. Oya M, Mikami S, Mizuno R, Marumo K, Mukai M, Murai M (2005) C-jun activation in acquired cystic kidney disease and renal cell carcinoma. J Urol 174:726

127. Rioux-Leclercq NC, Epstein JI (2003) Renal cell carcinoma with intratumoral calcium oxalate crystal deposition in patients with acquired cystic disease of the kidney. Arch Pathol Lab Med 127:E89–92

128. Sule N, Yakupoglu U, Shen SS, Krishnan B, Yang G, Lerner S, Sheikh-Hamad D, Truong LD (2005) Calcium oxalate deposition in renal cell carcinoma associated with acquired cystic kidney disease: a comprehensive study. Am J Surg Pathol 29:443–451

129. Bernstein J, Evan AP, Gardner KDJ (1987) Epithelial hyperplasia in human polycystic kidney diseases: its role in pathogenesis and risk of neoplasia. Am J Pathol 129:92–101

130. Knudson AGJ (1987) A two-mutation model for human cancer. Adv Viral Oncol 7:1–17

131. Gardner KDJ (1988) Cystic kidneys. Kidney Int 33:610–621

132. Ishikawa I, Saito Y, Nakazawa T, Shiroma K, Suzuki K (1998) Local recurrence of renal cell carcinoma and acquired cysts 10 years after tumour nephrectomy. Nephrol Dial Transplant 13:3236–3239

Index

Made in the USA
Monee, IL
07 July 2026